GUMPTIONADE

GUMPTIONADE℠

The Booster for Your Self-Improvement Plan

Robert B. O'Connor

Publisher's Cataloging-in-Publication data
O'Connor, Robert Baitsell.
Gumptionade : the booster for your self-improvement plan / Robert B. O'Connor.
pages cm
ISBN 978-0-9908884-1-3
Includes index and bibliographical references.

1. Self-actualization (Psychology). 2. Success. 3. Conduct of life. 4. Weight
loss. 5. Happiness. 6. Self-help techniques. I. Title.

BF637.S4 O362 2016

158.1 –dc23   2014958433

www.gumptionade.com
1 2 3 4 5 6 7 8 9
Printed in the United States of America on acid-free paper
Interior design by Typeflow
FIRST EDITION

For Doralina

Perhaps the most
valuable result of all
education is the ability
to make yourself do the
thing you have to do,
when it ought to be done,
whether you like it or not.

THOMAS HUXLEY

GUMPTIONWORK
Worksheets

Fundamentals of *Gumptionade*
(bold = section summary)

CONTENTS

Bonus *Gumptionade* material — including
deleted sections, interactive worksheets,
and a poster of Thomas Huxley's
"the most valuable result of all education"
quote — is available free at
www.gumptionade.com/readers-bonus.

INTRODUCTION

My father kept a poster on his dresser. Mounted on cardboard, it was the size of a file folder. He must have seen it every day. The poster was a quote from Thomas Huxley, a nineteenth-century British biologist. Tan words on a brown background: "Perhaps the most valuable result of all education is the ability to make yourself do the thing you have to do, when it ought to be done, whether you like it or not."

Huxley was self-taught. The education he was referring to was probably not four years at King's College, Cambridge. I believe his words were both inspiration and scourge for my father. They have been that for me.

I broke down in June of 2004. The nearest causes were a second failed marriage and a business that was breached and sinking, my income and fragile ego handcuffed to the oars.

I had a month of harrowing anxiety, perfect insomnia, and despair. The only thing I did with any conviction was journal and hope for the return of my right mind. That was the beginning of *Gumptionade*.

I wrote about Huxley's words and the opportunities I had missed to do what needed to be done. I recalled the concept of gumption in Robert Pirsig's *Zen and the Art of Motorcycle Maintenance*.

Gumption is an old-timey word for spunk and common sense. People with gumption — often seemingly unsophisticated characters who happen to be quite wise — are staples of folklore the world over.

This role was played to great effect by the American humorist Will Rogers: "Why don't they pass a constitutional amendment prohibiting anybody from learning anything? If it works as good as Prohibition did, in five years we will have the smartest people on Earth."

Sheriff Andy Taylor of the 1960s television comedy *The Andy Griffith Show* had gumption. His unassuming manner disguised a courageous and resourceful master of human nature who protected his eccentric community of Mayberry, North Carolina. This included protecting the self-esteem of Barney Fife, his incompetent and superbly grandiose deputy.

Pirsig set out a different but — I think — complementary definition of gumption: "Psychic gasoline." Fuel for getting work done. "If you are going to repair a motorcycle," he wrote about life, including life with a motorcycle, "an adequate supply of gumption is the first and most important tool."

Huxley's "most valuable result of all education" combined in my mind with Pirsig's "psychic gasoline." Both described the power to do the thing we have to do, when it ought to be done, whether we like it or not. I began to call that power gumption.

I was an embarrassment to myself when I began to write

Gumptionade. I had not done what needed to be done, when it needed to be done. I was living with the consequences.

I wasn't alone. Americans waste billions of dollars and hours each year on self-improvement plans and products. We try and fail to lose weight, get organized, exercise regularly, be a better spouse, a better parent, save for the future, or reach other important goals.

We give up and then, often around the beginning of the year, we read another book, try another plan, buy another product. And we fail again. We lose ground while we look for answers in the wrong places.

Worst of all, we feel bad about ourselves. We know that we are the main barrier to our own progress. We know what needs to be done. We cannot make ourselves do it. We cannot govern ourselves reasonably.

I recovered my mental health. I started a tiny business that paid my bills and I strengthened my ties with family and friends. I wrote this book. I learned how to do what needed to be done, when it needed to be done. Not all the time, but often enough.

Gumptionade is an essay expressing a primary idea: Your happiness depends largely on what you choose to do — or not do — with the cards life deals you. Gumption is the power to play your hand well, to do what needs to be done when it needs to be done. This is the power to make better choices.

Gumption is courage, resourcefulness, and common sense in harness together. These are attributes that I strengthened.

These are attributes that you can strengthen. You may already have a plan to do better — perhaps a diet, a workout routine, or a strategy to build your wealth. *Gumptionade* is a booster for your plan.

If you don't have a plan to do better, to be more than you are now, read *Gumptionade* before you make one. The worksheets alone will improve your thinking, particularly: "How to Be Less Wrong: A Checklist for Making Better Decisions."

I hope you find *Gumptionade* helpful. I hope it makes you smile a time or two. Life is sometimes grand, sometimes tragic, and often perfectly ridiculous. Let's laugh together at the ridiculous parts, so we get our money's worth from living through them.

Onward.

I

GUMPTION

Chapter 1

BUCKETS OF GUMPTION

Houston, we've had a problem.

Jim Lovell, astronaut

O N THE SECOND DAY OF ROCKETING toward the moon at two thousand miles per hour, Apollo 13 suffered a catastrophic explosion of oxygen tank number 2. "We had a pretty loud bang," Commander Lovell radioed to Mission Control.

Like blood from a wound, glowing vapor gathered around the spacecraft as oxygen poured out. Oxygen needed for breathing. Oxygen needed to generate the power to fly the ship at all, let alone fly it back to Earth. Apollo 13 and the three souls inside began to drift out of control.

Their mission was no longer lunar exploration but survival. The fastest way home required three days of flying. The fastest way home required three days of breathing.

The world looked up at the sky in wonder and worry. Then the gaze shifted to NASA's Manned Spacecraft Center in Houston. Everyone there looked to Apollo 13 Flight Director

Gene Kranz. He alone was responsible for all efforts to prevent three colleagues he knew and liked from asphyxiating and floating off into space forever.

After data confirmed the situation was dire, Flight Director Kranz asserted his authority and responsibility. He issued three orders:

1. Keep cool,
2. Solve the problem, and
3. Let's not make the situation any worse by guessing.

Kranz called for courage, resourcefulness, and common sense in harness together. That is to say, he called for gumption.

Courage: The team on the ground and in space became too busy interpreting data and exploring options to panic. *Common sense*: Neither the astronauts nor Mission Control did anything to make the desperate situation worse. *Resourcefulness*: They made astonishing use of the limited means at hand.

The three astronauts left the command module and powered it down to save electricity for the flight back. The attached lunar lander became their lifeboat. To conserve power and water, Apollo 13 switched to the guidance system designed for landing on the moon. Flight trajectory was changed to spare the damaged engines — the moon's gravity would slingshot the spacecraft back toward Earth.

Engineers on the ground helped the astronauts create a lifesaving device for removing carbon dioxide from the lunar lander's air supply, using a space suit air hose as a filter holder. They also invented a protocol for in-flight power-up of the command module section of the spacecraft.

About one hour before the end of the sixth day of traveling, Apollo 13 landed safely in the South Pacific. All hands on board had been saved by gumption: courage, resourcefulness, and common sense ("Let's not make the situation any worse by guessing").

Instead of stranded astronauts, perhaps you need to recover a healthy weight, or financial stability, or your momentum in life, or just plain your self-respect. You wouldn't be reading this if you didn't want to do better, to be more than you are now, to make real and lasting change.

"My name is Ann and I am an alcoholic," said a stylishly dressed sixty-year-old woman to a group of other female alcoholics and drug addicts. In prison.

That may or may not have been news to them. This visitor, with her clear blue eyes, her scarlet lipstick, and her flamboyant silver bouffant, was the most prominent recovering alcoholic in the state of Texas. What with her being governor.

Perhaps the prisoners wondered just how Ann Richards, a liberal, Democrat, divorced female alcoholic got herself elected governor of the great and conservative state of Texas.

Courage, resourcefulness, and common sense, that's how. Ann Richards had buckets of gumption. She took herself from full-time homemaker raising four children to political campaign volunteer, to commissioner of Travis County, to Texas state treasurer, to governor.

Ann Richards was resourceful. She created her first political platform out of whole cloth, helping to found the North Dallas Democratic Women in the early 1960s. She became a formidable political operative statewide, working to elect progressives to the state legislature and training women candidates. Bright, beautiful, caring, painstaking, and creative, Ann Richards brought a lot to the party.

She also brought a dependency on alcohol. That stopped on a Sunday morning in 1980 when, as she said, her "dear and closest friends and family, some of my finest drinking companions among them," intervened in her life. They told her how out of control her drinking was.

"We had to do it!" said one of her friends. "Just the driving was insane, with Ann roaring around the narrow roads up in those hills." When elected governor of Texas in 1990, Ann Richards had not taken a drink for over ten years.

She drank for the same reason most people do: Drinking changed how she felt about herself. Alcohol made her feel attractive, smart, and funny. It eased her worries and relaxed her drive to make things — to be — perfect: "You know what alcohol does, what it does is anesthetize you. You don't have to feel bad when you're drunk. Some people can have a couple of drinks and stop. With me there was no stopping...But that didn't bother me, 'cause everyone I ran with drank; I wasn't different."

On intervention day in 1980, she felt different. She felt afraid: "I was a public person. There was no way I could survive it." But Ann Richards was courageous. She returned from a month in rehab determined to be open and honest about her alcoholism. She acted on that decision one year later, during her successful campaign for state treasurer. Texas voters were not required to guess about her drinking.

It's common sense to be frugal. The first female Texas state treasurer was frugal with the taxpayers' money. Ann Richards streamlined her department and generated more nontax revenue for the state than all previous treasurers combined. Reelected in 1986, she was the first woman in Texas to serve two consecutive terms in statewide office.

Ann Richards's keynote address to the 1988 Democratic National Convention is one of the best-remembered speeches of the past fifty years. Her Waco twang magnified her criticism of the Reagan administration and the presumptive Republican presidential nominee: "I'm delighted to be here with you this evening, because after listening to George Bush all these years, I figured you needed to know what a real Texas accent sounds like...Poor George, he can't help it. He was born with a silver foot in his mouth."

During her single term as governor, Richards performed the Herculean task of cleaning up the notoriously backward Texas state bureaucracy, parts of which were under court order. This included significant reforms to the prison system. She added capacity and programs to treat drug and alcohol addiction.

She also attended AA meetings, gave public talks about her recovery, and wrote hundreds of personal notes to fellow alcoholics.

Ann Richards was the first governor to name significant numbers of minorities and women to key roles in Texas government, including the first black and the first female Texas Rangers (real Texas Rangers).

Oil was eight dollars a barrel when Ann Richards became governor. Her administration put programs in place that allowed the sputtering Texas economy to benefit from the boom that occurred years later.

She was a liberal Democrat in the early years of the conservative Republican resurgence in the South. She was defeated for reelection as governor in 1994 by George W. Bush, a very different kind of native Texan ex-drinker.

Gone now, Ann Richards remains a legend among Texas progressives, an inspiration to leadership-oriented women and girls nationwide, and a touchstone for those seeking to achieve or maintain sobriety.

The closing words of her speech at the Celebration of Recovery in Dallas in 1995 seem a fitting farewell from a person with buckets of gumption: "Take heart. We're all better than we think we are."

You are better than you think you are. But you need a sound plan — a good process — to *do* better. Sound plans are usually simple but rarely easy. You may already have one.

This book is a booster for your self-improvement plan, like Oxyclean™ is a booster for laundry detergent. It makes a good process work better.

Gumptionade will prepare you for what I call "Day Four,"

the moment when your beautiful plan comes in contact with reality. The reality of just how difficult it is to make real and lasting change.

You'll need gumption on Day Four, when your enthusiasm is gone and your real suffering arrives. You'll need courage, resourcefulness, and common sense.

The Oakland Athletics are astonishing. With nearly the lowest payroll in major league baseball, they win nearly the most games. The A's have been consistently better than larger-market teams with larger budgets. Perhaps you know of their general manager, Billy Beane. Perhaps you read Michael Lewis's brilliant *Moneyball* or saw the movie. The A's are a story about gumption: courage, resourcefulness, and common sense applied to the business of professional baseball.

Billy Beane became general manager a few months before the 1998 season. Since then, the A's have won 1,484 baseball games at a cost of $570,000 per win. Every other team in the major leagues paid more per win. The New York Mets paid twice as much.

How did the A's do it? By defying the accepted wisdom of the baseball establishment. By using a common sense, fact-based strategy for winning baseball games.

A new star had appeared in the baseball sky in 1998. Like most revolutionary things, it appeared in humble guise. That star was sabermetrics, "the search for objective knowledge about baseball." Invented by baseball fans, sabermetrics used a creative, fact-based approach to evaluate the effectiveness of individual ballplayers in producing runs.

Other major league teams did not see this new star. They saw only the status quo, the traditional beliefs about evaluating players.

Don't be surprised. Great leaps forward usually come from the margins: a garage in Los Altos (Jobs and Wozniak); Robbin Island (Mandela); Stratford-Upon-Avon (Shakespeare); a trading settlement in northern Arabia (Muhammad); the dusty town of Nazareth (Jesus Christ). Sabermetrics was just an entertaining diversion for a few high I.Q. baseball fans — until it fundamentally changed the axioms of assembling a major league team.

Wandering in the western desert of the American League, Billy Beane looked up to the heavens and saw sabermetrics. His eye filled with light. He could recognize new facts about excellence on the baseball field. He had options. The A's stopped guessing about the most cost-efficient way to score runs.

Baseball players who maintain high batting averages contribute heavily to the total runs scored by their teams. A high batting average is vivid — easy to see, and easy to understand. Players who maintain high batting averages are expensive. Everybody knows who they are and what they can do. What everybody knows isn't worth knowing.

Beane saw the new fact revealed by sabermetrics: Something else is as reliable as batting average in predicting the contribution of a player to runs scored. This thing is called "on-base percentage."

Batting average is calculated by dividing the number of hits a player makes by their number of chances at bat. This formula, developed in the nineteenth century, does not count a base on balls — a walk — as either a hit or an at bat.

Every kid who ever played baseball was told that a walk is as good as a hit. It's common sense: like a hit, a walk puts a potential run on base.

But when hiring players, major league baseball teams ignored that common sense. A walk seemed weak; they'd take it, sure, but they wouldn't count it. On-base percentage, which calculated walks as well as hits, was uninspiring to them.

Not to Billy Beane. He saw that some players who lacked the expensive attribute of a high batting average did have a high on-base percentage. They drew a lot of walks. Sabermetrics proved that these players manufactured lots of runs for their teams.

They manufactured these runs at a low cost as well, because this type of player was undervalued. Players who got a lot of walks relative to hits were excellent players the Oakland A's could actually afford.

The cost to Billy Beane of using this knowledge was the discomfort of hiring players who did not fit the status quo. Batting average, home runs, and even athleticism were not important considerations for the A's. Player selection was about on-base percentage. Radical.

It's not easy to go against the status quo. Do things the accepted way and fail, and at least you can say you did what

everybody does. But ignore conventional wisdom and fail —
then it's your fault. You may not get another job in major
league baseball. Bearing that risk takes courage.

Beane and his A's were first ignored, then mocked, then criticized for their approach to winning. Then widely copied. In
baseball, and then in other professional sports.

Extracting knowledge from failure is resourceful. Billy Beane
knew failure in baseball. He had played the game at a high
level and was selected by the New York Mets (irony) in the
first round of the 1980 amateur draft (the year Ann Richards
got sober).

He had the build, the speed, the batting average, and the
home run swing. Billy Beane was also handsome. A can't-miss
major league star.

Can't miss did miss. Billy Beane spent several years roam-
ing through Tidewater, Toledo, Tacoma, and other border-
lands of professional baseball. He collected only eleven walks
from his 301 total major league at-bats. His on-base percentage was terrible.

Billy Beane paid attention to the facts of his own failure, to
the fact that those whom the establishment values are not the
only ones with value. He prepared himself to use sabermetrics
before he knew such a thing existed.

We *have a flight director* with a crippled spaceship halfway to the moon, a recovering alcoholic running for public office, a baseball general manager needing to win big on a small budget. Interesting. But what do they mean for *your* plan to be better, to do what needs to be done?

They can teach you about gumption. Gene Kranz, Ann Richards, and Billy Beane were resourceful. They used the means at hand to give themselves a chance. They had common sense — they focused on knowing, not guessing. On facts. They bore their risks with courage. That's what you need. That's what I need. That's gumption.

Let's proceed for a closer look at the three attributes of gumption — after a slight detour for an exercise you can do now.

Complete the work sheet that follows, if you please, to see how much gumption you already have.

GUMPTIONWORK

Personal Gumption Appraisal

You can do this better online:
www.gumptionade.com/measure-your-gumption

Do you have buckets of gumption or teaspoons? This exercise is designed to give you some idea. Answer the questions below and tally up your score at the end.

If a question doesn't seem to apply to you, just do your best to interpret it in a way that does apply. If you live in New York and have never owned a car, for example, just make an honest guess as to how things would be if you *did* own a car. We are trying to be directional here, not precise.

Courage

	TRUE 2 POINTS	FALSE 0 POINTS
I can be physically uncomfortable without making the people around me miserable.	☐	☐
I can laugh at myself.	☐	☐
I have steered into a skid.	☐	☐
I can remove a spider from my home without spraying or squashing it.	☐	☐
I have an emergency plan.	☐	☐
I will haggle over a price.	☐	☐
I will change a poopy diaper.	☐	☐
I don't get upset when someone insults me.	☐	☐
I have not procrastinated on a truly important task in over a year.	☐	☐

Continued...

12

GUMPTIONWORK

Courage, cont'd	TRUE 2 POINTS	FALSE 0 POINTS
I spoke my honest disagreement to someone more powerful than me in the last six months.	☐	☐
I will talk respectfully to anyone, but I will not be hustled.	☐	☐
I have asked someone way out of my league on a date.	☐	☐
I admitted I was wrong about something important in the past three months.	☐	☐
I was calm under fire in the last year.	☐	☐
I stopped and helped a stranger in the past six months.	☐	☐
I have lost a lot of weight and kept it off for at least a year, or quit smoking for at least a year, or got and stayed sober. *Bonus: 6 points for a true answer on this question*	☐	☐

COURAGE SCORE: _____

Resourcefulness

	TRUE 2 POINTS	FALSE 0 POINTS
I can change a tire.	☐	☐
I have used at least two of the following items in the past year: WD-40, duct tape, a screwdriver, compost, needle and thread, shoe trees, stain remover, steel wool, an old T-shirt (as something other than clothing).	☐	☐
I know CPR.	☐	☐
I put on a sweater before I turn up the heat.	☐	☐
I get enough sleep.	☐	☐
I ask questions when I don't understand.	☐	☐
I know where my money goes.	☐	☐
I get things in writing and I put them in writing.	☐	☐

Continued...

GUMPTIONWORK

Resourcefulness, cont'd	TRUE 2 POINTS	FALSE 0 POINTS
When the computer won't work, I try to fix the problem for at least ten minutes before I give up and call someone.	☐	☐
I used a thesaurus in the past month.	☐	☐
I return things for refunds.	☐	☐
I have a spare key and I know where it is.	☐	☐
I can prepare a decent meal from simple ingredients.	☐	☐
I don't always follow the directions, but I always read them.	☐	☐
I stock up on the boring stuff when I meet a good price.	☐	☐
I was inspired by something I read in the last year.	☐	☐

RESOURCEFULNESS SCORE: _____

Common sense

	TRUE 2 POINTS	FALSE 0 POINTS
I always wear a seat belt.	☐	☐
I have not had too much to drink for at least three years.	☐	☐
I am skeptical of politicians, business leaders, and church officials — even the ones I like.	☐	☐
I do not smoke.	☐	☐
I am saving about enough for my retirement.	☐	☐
I get about enough exercise.	☐	☐
I have not had unsafe sex for over three years.	☐	☐
I paid less than fifty dollars in overdraft fees in the last three years.	☐	☐
I am not obese.	☐	☐

Continued...

GUMPTIONWORK

Common sense, cont'd	TRUE 2 POINTS	FALSE 0 POINTS
I haven't gotten a speeding ticket in the last five years.	☐	☐
I have paid less than fifty dollars in credit card interest in the last three years.	☐	☐
I don't get into arguments with strangers.	☐	☐
I floss.	☐	☐
I have not made an impulse purchase greater than one hundred dollars for at least three years.	☐	☐
I do not believe in any of the following: painless dentistry, easy weight loss, retail therapy, exact estimates, committee action, gourmet pet food.	☐	☐
My car is paid for.	☐	☐

COMMON SENSE SCORE: _____

GUMPTION SCORE:
(COURAGE + RESOURCEFULNESS + COMMON SENSE)
☐

Your Gumption

80–100 points	60–79 points	Under 60 points
Buckets of Gumption	Just Enough Gumption	Insufficient Gumption

Chapter 2

GUMPTION IS COURAGE

"Follow me boys, bayonets forward."

COLONEL JOSHUA CHAMBERLAIN
(TO HIS TWENTIETH MAINE AT GETTYSBURG, LOW
ON AMMUNITION AND FACING A FOURTH CHARGE
BY THE GALLANT FIFTEENTH ALABAMA)

G UMPTION IS COURAGE, RESOURCEFUL-
ness, and common sense. We'll start our review of
these attributes with courage, because resourcefulness and common sense—when you really need them—don't
work well without courage. Courage is characterized by knowing, daring, and bearing (fortitude).

Quincy Magoo, Rutgers class of 1903, is the extremely
nearsighted central character of the TV cartoon *The Famous
Adventures of Mr. Magoo*. The jokes center around the misun-
derstandings and near disasters caused by his refusal to recognize his poor vision. Magoo drives his yellow Model T on top
of the locomotive, through the cow barn, and onto the roller-
coaster track. He can't be called courageous—he never sees
the risks he is taking.

Part of courage is knowing. Knowing when to be afraid and when not to be. Knowing what you risk.

In *Fooled by Randomness*, Nassim Taleb writes about some Magoos he met on Wall Street. These were traders whose dazzling short-term success blinded them to the giant risks they were taking with their companies' money and their own careers.

Taleb sees no problem with taking big risks in exchange for big rewards (although that's not how *he* got rich), provided one does not believe or pretend that the risk is trivial. But with these Wall Street Magoos, "There was no courage in their taking such risks, just ignorance."

Sapere aude: Dare to know. Part of courage. Part of gumption.

MEN WANTED
for hazardous journey, small wages, bitter cold, long months of complete darkness, constant danger, safe return doubtful, honor and recognition in case of success.
Ernest Shackleton   4 Burlington st.

The legendary newspaper advertisement for Ernest Shackleton's 1914 expedition to Antarctica.

Thanks to press coverage and word of mouth, Ernest Shackleton received many applications to join his trans-Antarctic expedition in 1914. Many applicants were Magoos, ignorant of the risks involved.

The crew members selected for the voyage were not. They

knew the risks: most had extensive experience at sea. Several
had been members of previous Antarctic expeditions, parts of
which had been harrowing. They dared.

They were prepared when risk turned into calamity. Their
wooden ship, *Endurance*, became trapped in an ice floe, broke
up in the spring thaw, and sank. With the expedition now
camped on floating ice, the mission changed from exploration to survival.

Shackleton and five others sailed a lifeboat eight hundred
miles through stormy seas to the bottom of desolate South
Georgia Island. They hiked thirty-two miles north to a whal-
ing station. (Thereby making the first known overland cross-
ing of the Allardyce mountain range.) They organized a rescue
party there and retrieved the rest of their crew.

There are uncertainties in every venture. But uncertainty
can be translated into risk. Only when risk is understood can
there be daring, can there be courage. Without understanding risk, you are a Magoo.

To go to plant your flag on the bottom of the world is to
dare. To dare is also to challenge your own beliefs, those of
your family, your industry, your religion, your society. To dare
is to accept the risk of misery on the path to being more than
you are now.

Weight-bearing capacity — grace under pressure — is also part
of courage. Fortitude (from the Latin word for strong) allows
you to bear discomfort.

That discomfort can come from fear, frustration, embarrassment, impatience, or physical pain. The heaviest weight to be borne is often not the discomfort itself but the anticipation of it. (How often have you said to yourself, "Now that wasn't so bad, was it?")

It takes fortitude to deny impulses — the impulse to blurt out your opinions, to break your diet, to get high, to scream at your child, to skip that workout. It takes fortitude to veto any number of ideas that seem so right in the moment and so wrong in the sober light of dawn. It takes fortitude to stand fast.

Julia Hill climbed a redwood in Northern California's Humboldt County one December day in 1997. She planned to use her body to protect the centuries-old tree from being logged by its owner, Pacific Lumber Company.

She was not, as she had expected, going to be tree sitting (previous world record: one hundred days). She was going to be tree *living*. On a twelve-foot-by-twelve-foot platform, 180 feet above the ground. Having grown up traveling the United States in a trailer with her evangelist father and the rest of her family, Julia was prepared for tight spaces.

Climbing a redwood tree takes daring. *Living* in a redwood tree takes fortitude. That area of Northern California is wet and windy. Winter temperatures routinely go below freezing. At 180 feet the weather is more severe. More severe than that is the effect of gravity on a human being falling from that height.

Hill bore the discomfort of freezing rain, forty-mile-per-hour winds, and insomnia-inducing nocturnal squirrels. She was not moved by death threats from irate loggers, a ten-day siege by Pacific Lumber security guards, or an existential confrontation with the Chinook helicopter sent to deafen her with engine noise and blow her out of the tree with winds from twin sixty-foot rotors.

Julia Hill remained steadfast. She learned not to wash the sap off her feet in order to maintain traction on the branches. She would not be moved.

She climbed down in 1999. In return, Pacific Lumber agreed to spare her tree and all redwoods within two hundred feet of it. Fortitude. Courage.

Physical courage is the willingness to bear the risk of suffering physical pain. Moral courage is the willingness to bear the risk of suffering emotional pain, including disapproval and discouragement. Emotional pain may come from others or it may come from resisting the force of your own bad habits.

Recovering a crippled spacecraft from the void of outer space, recovering yourself from addiction, challenging the status quo of your industry, or risking your life to protect redwoods — all require courage.

So do less dramatic actions, such as sticking to a diet, exercising when you don't care to, being gentle with people when you are angry, admitting you were wrong, and just plain being present and accounted for every day.

Courage is fundamental to doing what needs to be done, when it needs to be done. But courage alone is not enough. You have to have common sense and resourcefulness in harness with it.

Chapter 3

GUMPTION IS RESOURCEFULNESS

We don't need more strength or more
ability or greater opportunity. What
we need is to use what we have.

—Basil Walsh

S TEVE JOBS GOT A TOUR OF XEROX'S PALO
Alto Research Center (PARC) in late 1979. Part of the
tour was a demonstration of the Alto, a prototype personal computer running point-and-click software, using a
device called a mouse.

Jobs: "It was like a veil being lifted from my eyes. I could see
what the future of computing was destined to be."

Resourcefulness, the knack for finding ways to get things
done, is the second part of gumption. Resourcefulness is characterized by vision — the ability to see the means at hand —
creativity, and WhoHowness. (Your author has invented that
word to name the indispensable skill of knowing who, how,
and when to ask for help.)

Apple was also working on an easy-to-use small computer. At PARC, Jobs saw that Xerox had solved many of the problems Apple's engineers were struggling with. Just seeing that the problems could be solved was the means at hand for Apple to solve them too.

Apple introduced the Mac in 1984, priced for the mass consumer audience. Xerox never made a commercially successful computer. Jobs saw what Xerox could not because:

1. He was the only Steve Jobs in the room, and
2. His decision frame was broader: "They were copier-heads who had no clue what a computer could do," he told his biographer. Said more politely, Xerox lacked the experience Jobs got from selling the Apple I and II to consumers.

Xerox thought they could sell thousands of computers to businesses already using computers. Jobs looked at their Alto and saw the means at hand to sell millions of computers to consumers who did not yet own one. His vision made Apple more resourceful than Xerox. Apple had more gumption.

Physician John Snow invented epidemiology during the terrifying London cholera outbreak of 1854. He went door to door in Soho, the most affected area, counting the number of people in each house who had been sickened. He then drew a map of the neighborhood, showing the number *and location* of confirmed cholera cases.

There were no public water lines. Households obtained their drinking water from pumps scattered around the city. Water from Soho's Broad Street pump was considered superior. This was before germ theory, but not before germs.

Snow's map gave him vision. He saw the correlation between cholera cases and households using the Broad Street pump. He saw microbes without the benefit of a microscope. He saw cholera moving invisibly through water. This contradicted leading scientists, who believed that cholera and other urban epidemics were caused by "miasmas," bad air found in densely populated areas.

Snow convinced the local council to remove the handle on the Broad Street pump. He subsequently discovered that

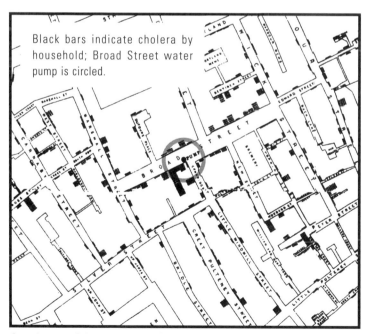

Black bars indicate cholera by household; Broad Street water pump is circled.

Snow's map of the 1854 Broad Street cholera outbreak in London provided visual evidence in the era before germ theory.

its water had been poisoned by sewage from a nearby household cesspit.

John Snow saw the footprint of cholera and translated it into statistical fact, the means at hand to end the outbreak. Vision. Resourcefulness. Gumption.

Public health medicine in London in the 1850s was practiced under conditions of uncertainty and unpredictability—in what is now called a low-validity environment. An example in our own time is online dating. It's wise to develop simple formulas for decision making in low-validity environments. In London's cholera epidemic, it was the households' source of drinking water and cases of cholera. In online dating, it's age, education, and income.

It's resourceful to draw a map. Dr. Snow drew a paper map of cholera's footprint. Steve Jobs carried a mental map of a mass consumer market that did not yet exist. Billy Beane took sabermetrics and mapped undervalued baseball players. All three used the means at hand to see what others could not.

The baseball establishment, Xerox, and the leading scientists of Victorian England had narrower vision. They did not recognize the new facts. They were not resourceful. They lacked gumption.

Improve your own vision. Look for facts about yourself. Map the things that you do.

Sam John Hopkins of Centerville, Texas, wanted a guitar, but was too poor to buy one. He solved his problem by using the means at hand: a cigar box, scrap wood, wire, and glue. That is how Lightnin' Hopkins got a guitar. Creative use of the means at hand is resourcefulness.

How will you stay alive after you've used up the lithium hydroxide air filters that fit the round canister in the Apollo 13 lunar lander — now your lifeboat? You will asphyxiate if you can't remove carbon dioxide from your atmosphere, but your remaining air filters fit only the command module's square canister. You proceed to make creative use of the means at hand. You invent "an adapter for the square command module canister from cardboard, a plastic bag, a sock, and a hose from one of the crew's pressure suits." Creative use of the means at hand.

How can the German owner of a Polish factory save his Jewish employees from concentration camps? *Schindlerjuden* is how.

Oskar Schindler made astonishing use of his means at hand during World War II — an industrial smelter, metal oxides, bribes, falsified records, scotch, black market dealings, and above all salesmanship — to create a "war effort essential" enamelware production facility. Employees of such a factory could be hidden in plain sight.

What do you do when you are building the University of Virginia and need to know where to put paved pathways? Thomas Jefferson instructed the builders to wait a couple of years and then pave the trails people made in the grass as they walked from where they were to where they wanted to go. He used the means at hand — the student body — to make a map.

Resourceful people know who, how, and *when* to ask for help. WhoHowness is fundamental to Alcoholics Anonymous. Getting and giving help is baked into the program through regular meetings with other alcoholics.

Galileo Galilei had help proving the earth was not the center of the universe. As explained by the writer Adam Gopnick, he knew who and how to ask for help:

> Galileo soon began to have doubts about this [heliocentric] orthodoxy, which he aired in conversation with friends and then in correspondence with other natural philosophers in Europe, particularly the great German astronomer Johannes Kepler.

About 150 years later, a fundamental truth was unveiled in the new world. The Declaration of Independence contains one of the most important ideas ever put into words:

> We hold these truths to be self-evident, that all men are created equal, that they are endowed by their Creator with certain unalienable Rights, that among these are Life, Liberty and the pursuit of Happiness.

The author was Thomas Jefferson. John Adams, Benjamin Franklin, Roger Sherman of Connecticut, and Robert Livingston of New York reviewed his drafts and suggested improvements. The Continental Congress made its own revisions before adopting the document on July 4, 1776. Jefferson had more WhoHowness than he wanted. Nonetheless, something astonishing emerged.

A *bicycle shop co-owner wrote to* the Smithsonian Institution in 1899. Wilbur Wright wanted to know how the experts there could help him understand the science of flight.

He then used the ideas and experiments of Leonardo da Vinci (sixteenth-century studies of bird flight), nineteenth-century aerodynamics studies of Sir George Cayley, and the experiments and models of contemporary aeronautics pioneers.

The advances made by others in wing design and engine science freed Wright to focus on pilot control, the third aspect of "the flying problem." Human-controlled flight had a high incidence of crash landing and pilot death. What was lacking, what was crucial, was stability.

There were many reasons that within four years Wilbur Wright was able to invent the three-axis control (still standard for fixed-wing aircraft) and then the first successful engine-powered airplane. Intelligence and drive were two of these, but insufficient by themselves. WhoHowness — resourcefulness — was fundamental. One resource was a brother named Orville.

Other famous demonstrators of WhoHowness include:

1. Rosalind Franklin, James Watson, and Francis Crick, who mapped the structure of DNA
2. John Lennon and Paul McCartney, one of the best songwriting teams ever
3. William Procter and James Gamble (did I mention I once worked at a soap company?)
4. Cassius Clay and Angelo Dundee, co-creators of the boxing genius Muhammad Ali

WhoHowness: How to
Ask a Bigshot for Help

I awoke one morning during my senior year at Kenyon College and realized I would not join the Marines upon graduation, as I had thought. I needed to line up a civilian job.

The daughter of the president of Procter & Gamble was a classmate. As a result, P&G sent a recruiter from their renowned marketing department to our college. I learned what P&G marketing was like from a roommate's older brother, a brand assistant there. His tales of the job interested me, especially the princely starting salary.

He also told me about the caliber of applicants I would compete against: Harvard Business School graduates, West Point–trained officers with five years' active duty, and student body presidents from large universities (which he had been). Generally speaking, a pool of outstanding men and women with accomplishments I lacked.

Aren't we always attracted to groups that will not have us? I submitted my résumé. Based on the strength of that document, P&G declined to schedule an interview. Now *that* I did not expect. I was miffed.

I did two things. I woke at 6:00 a.m. to sign up for a first-come-first-served open interview slot. Then I wrote a letter to John Smale, the president of P&G—to whom I was unknown—to ask for his help. That was ambitious WhoHowness, but really, what did I have to lose?

I wrote to him on stationary purchased at the college bookstore. Kenyon stationary. Recall the man's daughter was my classmate (it's resourceful to take your luck). That got me past his secretary. I also took care to make it the best letter I could write about myself. My favorite subject.

John Smale sent it to the Procter & Gamble Personnel Department with a note in the top right-hand corner: "I don't know who the hell this guy is, but he can write a letter." That's all it takes. One week after graduation I was selling soap in Cincinnati (Scope, actually).

(A copy of my golden letter is available at www.gumptionade.com/ my-golden-letter.)

Doesn't it make you feel good to help someone? To share what you know? That's only human. Bigshots are human, too, even if they *are* busy humans.

Take courage. What have you got to lose? Yes, your ego will throb if you are ignored, but your ego can't give you the help you need.

Trust in God *and* tie up your camel. After P&G turned me down, I hustled for an open interview slot and wrote a Hail Mary letter to the CEO. Do *your* part.

Are you going to say something like "May I pick your brain?" or "Can we meet for coffee?" to a Bigshot you don't already know? Do *not* bring that weakness. Don't make a Bigshot guess: Ask for exactly the help you want.

Here's how I ended my letter to John Smale: "If my qualifications seem proper to you, I would appreciate your passing that information along to Sandy Moersdorf [the interviewer visiting Kenyon]." What could be simpler than that?

Anything you put in writing has to be perfect. And brief.

It is absurd to try to hurry a Bigshot because you have procrastinated. You want a favor, *and* you want them to scramble their schedule to do it for you? Fuhgeddaboudit.

Be gracious: Thank a Bigshot for their time. Thank a Bigshot if they help you. Verbally, if possible, but *always* in writing. I send a note on paper. I use a stamp. Sometimes I include a five-dollar Starbucks gift card, to buy that Bigshot a cup of coffee. Enough to make them notice you but too little to be an insulting attempt at quid pro quo. They'll give it to their secretary. By the way, most secretaries are Bigshots.

And if the Godfather asks your help in return one day? All you need to know is where and when.

5. Lucille Ball and Desi Arnaz, inventors of the TV situation comedy
6. Bill Gates and Paul Allen, founders of Microsoft, who made software more important than hardware

WhoHowness is always resourceful but sometimes difficult. Eight years after he became the second human to walk on the moon, Buzz Aldrin had fallen into depression and alcoholism. A sober Aldrin later said: "Recovery was not easy. Perhaps the most challenging turnaround was accepting the need for assistance and help."

Going against conventional thinking can be resourceful, but it is usually difficult. WhoHowness helps you bear up. As Nassim Taleb writes in *The Black Swan*, it is easier to be part of an ostracized group than to be ostracized by yourself. Just ask a Log Cabin Republican.

Vision, creativity, and WhoHowness will make you more resourceful. Resourcefulness and courage are fundamental to meeting the challenges of life. But they need adult supervision to become gumption. They need common sense.

Chapter 4

GUMPTION IS
COMMON SENSE

*"Philosophy is common
sense with big words."*

JAMES MADISON

THE THIRD PART OF GUMPTION IS GOVERN-
ing yourself reasonably: Common sense is characterized by logic, prudence, and curiosity.

Most of us often don't use logic nearly as often as we use
psycho-logic. Important decisions are driven by habit, intuition, and emotion. Sometimes we don't have enough common sense to take off our jeans before we iron them.

> *Errors using inadequate data are much
> less than those using no data at all.*
>
> CHARLES BABBAGE

It is logical to follow the advice of Flight Director Kranz: Don't
guess. Know.

- Correlation is not causation. I say, "Things
  started to go wrong after Sue took over.
  She's got to go." Logic asks: "What is it
  that Sue did or failed to do that created
  problems?"
- Circular reasoning is not logic. "I could lose
  this weight if I had the willpower" means
  "I could lose this weight if I could lose this
  weight."
- Beliefs are not necessarily facts. Many
  people believe the Bible is the literal word
  of God. They may be right, but "because it
  says so in the Bible" is not proof.
- Starting with false premises is just guessing.
  "I am going to wash my car today. Take an
  umbrella if you go out." Don't guess. Know.

In his book *Calculated Risks*, Gerd Gigerenzer provided a
basis for logically interpreting the results of AIDS testing in
the 1990s. Here is an illustration:

"The test shows you are HIV positive," says the nurse at the
clinic. "I am sorry to give you such bad news."

The (heroically) logical person responds with facts: "I am
heterosexual. I have never been promiscuous. I don't use
drugs. What are the chances of a false positive on this test for
someone with no known risk factors for AIDS?" (About one
in two, at that time.) Rather than accepting the bad news and
seeking the recommended treatment, or just giving up, logic
looks for the cause of such an unlikely diagnosis.

Common sense requires logical thinking.

Prudence: Living within one's means is more than a financial issue. Americans with high stress from debt problems have heart attacks at twice the rate of those reporting low debt-related stress. Correlation does not equal causation, but consider that the Americans who *died* from heart attacks caused by debt-related stress could not complete the survey. One of the benefits of frugality may be postponing your own funeral.

> *Annual income twenty pounds, annual expenditure nineteen and six, result happiness. Annual income twenty pounds, annual expenditure twenty pounds ought and six, result misery.*
>
> WILKINS MACAWBER, FROM *DAVID COPPERFIELD* BY CHARLES DICKENS

There is nothing wrong with five-dollar lattes, credit card interest, designer bags, Montblanc pens, overdraft charges, ninety-dollar face cream, grand cru wine, statement watches, car payments, Jimmy Choo shoes, or Fiji water. If you can afford them.

Ophthalmologic surgeons who perform six to eight semi-miraculous eye surgeries every weekday take home over a million dollars a year. For them, using Montblanc pens, collecting fine wine, sporting a Rolex, and carrying a big car payment are prudent. They can buy those things and still be frugal.

But the doctors need to avoid the mortgage on a penthouse in Manhattan, getting divorced, owning thoroughbred racehorses, or playing high-stakes baccarat at the Mandarin Oriental.

PRUDENCE RULES OF TEN

1. Wait ten seconds before speaking when angry.

2. Wait ten minutes before taking another helping.

3. Wait ten hours before you send that angry or risqué email.

4. Wait ten days before you make the big impulse purchase.

5. Wait ten weeks before you look for *any* improvements from your self-improvement plan.

6. Wait ten months before you scrap your plan.

Warren Buffett, on the other hand, could do all these things (he doesn't) and still be frugal. However, Mr. Buffett should not buy Portugal.

Peter likes drinking whiskey and eating steak. His father liked drinking whiskey and eating steak, and smoked Lucky Strikes to boot. Peter's father died of a heart attack at age fifty-nine.

Peter exercises regularly. He counts his drinks and he counts

his steaks. He does not smoke. Peter is prudent with his cardiovascular system.

Prudence is risk reduction by means of self-discipline (you
could say self-love). Prudence is the ability to reduce the threat
of future misery by doing what needs to be done when it needs
to be done. This usually causes short-term discomfort. Calories are counted, exercise is taken, cavities are filled, luxuries
postponed, insurance premiums paid, inappropriate flirtations
avoided, and uncomfortable but necessary conversations are
stumbled through.

Prudence with your money and your health reduces the
risk of future misery. Not a complex moral judgment. Common sense.

Curiosity: Theoretical physicist Richard Feynman was
appointed to the commission investigating the *Challenger*
space shuttle disaster (seven souls lost in an explosion caused
by a fuel tank leak).

> *Do not block the way of inquiry.*
> CHARLES SANDERS PEIRCE

"Feynman is becoming a real pain," said Chairman William
Rogers at one point. Of course he was. Feynman was curious.
Feynman was a scientist. He wanted *facts*.

The Rogers commission conducted many hours of hear-
ings and received many written reports. Two facts available to
members — and to NASA before the disaster — were:

1. The outside temperature at lift-off was much lower than for any previous shuttle launch, and

2. The rubber O-ring seals played a crucial role in preventing fuel tank leaks.

Feynman was curious: Had a connection between these two facts caused the disaster?

A piece of O-ring was passed around during expert testimony. Feynman cooled the sample in his glass of ice water and pinched it. It failed to spring back into shape. The commission saw that very cold O-rings lost flexibility. Inflexible O-rings could cause a fuel tank to leak. Smoking gun.

Feynman went on to uncover the fact that NASA misunderstood commonly accepted measures of risk, understating the chance of a shuttle disaster "to the point of fantasy."

Nobel laureate Richard Feynman was smarter than the other members of the Rogers commission. He was also more curious. He had more common sense. He had gumption.

Curiosity helps you bypass obstacles to clear thinking, including incentives to ignore unpleasant facts. NASA's obstacle that cold afternoon was "Go Fever," the top-down bias of a group toward consensus and forward movement without effective consideration of risk.

Here on Earth, money is the primary cause of bias. If you find yourself unsure about where someone is coming from, be curious and follow the money.

Let us say you are sixty years old and have significant left knee pain while walking. The orthopedic surgeon says you need a knee replacement ($40,000). The chiropractor recommends manipulation (full course, $1,700). The acupuncturist recommends needles in your leg (five sessions, $600). Pfizer recommends Celebrex ($150 for thirty pills). The manager of the GNC store recommends Instaflex Joint Support supplement ($69.99).

Why would they each have a different opinion about what is best for you? Follow the money.

Your family doctor recommends you take aspirin (ten cents per day) and lose weight (free). This option will not make her any money. This is the best thing to try first.

People with common sense are capable of analyzing so-called reasonable explanations. They are curious enough to notice when puzzling facts appear, and to look for an explanation.

At one time in human history conventional thinking held that the earth was flat. It certainly looked flat. Nonetheless, certain visible facts suggested other options to the curious.

Sailors noticed that a ship's hull disappeared before the mast when it was sailing away. Why would that be? They then noticed that they could see that entire ship again if they climbed high up in the rigging of their own vessel. What could account for such observations? The Greek philosopher Aristotle noticed that the shadow the earth casts on the moon during a lunar eclipse is always round, regardless of the angle of the

sun's light. Once you have seen that, and understood its signif-
icance, the fact that the earth is round is just common sense.

Isaac Newton was curious about why apples don't fall up.
Obviously a force pulled them downward. Since there seemed
to be no height at which it wouldn't operate, this force must
extend across vast distances — even so far as the moon. This
force — the force of gravity — was influencing the orbit of the
moon. This new fact gave Newton options for explaining the
movement of the planets.

The acquisition of wisdom is a curiosity-driven process of
updating common sense with observed facts and discovering
new options. When you have been curious enough to look at
on-base percentage, you have new options for explaining how
baseball games are won. Do not block the way of inquiry.

By now you know what gumption *is*: courage, resourcefulness,
and common sense in harness together. It is also important to
know what gumption *is not.*

Chapter 5

GUMPTION IS
NOT THIS

*I don't wait for moods. You
accomplish nothing if you do that.*

Pearl S. Buck

EVERY JANUARY 1ST WE BECOME INFATU-
ated with the idea of a new and improved version
of ourselves: the thin version, the organized version,
the fit version, the better parent version, the debt-free version.
As with any crush, our enthusiasm is effortless and exciting, a
temporary loss of balance. Instead of flowers and chocolate,
we treat our new love to frozen diet meals, gym memberships,
brightly colored storage containers, bee pollen, packs of nico-
tine gum, how-to books and videos.

This happy buying and trying soon plays itself out. We lack
the courage, resourcefulness, and common sense required for
lasting change.

Enthusiasm is not gumption. Enthusiasm is like good luck:

great when you have it, but outside of your control. You can *act* enthusiastic, but you can't make yourself *be* enthusiastic. You either are or you aren't. Indeed, a sign of gumption is doing the thing that needs to be done when you have no enthusiasm for it.

Unlike gumption, enthusiasm is dependent on context. In *Zen and the Art of Motorcycle Maintenance*, Robert Pirsig writes of things that halt progress for amateurs repairing motorcycles: the scraped knuckle, the bad light, the heat, the cold, the uncomfortable crouching, the leftover engine parts. If you are trying to repair *yourself*, these might be a bad day at work, loneliness, boredom, hunger, insomnia, and family holidays.

Physical discomfort reduces enthusiasm. Emotional discomfort reduces enthusiasm. Mistakes reduce enthusiasm. None of these things reduce gumption, which is not dependent on context.

Gumption has courage. Courage helps you bear the suffering required to move forward without the tail winds of enthusiasm. For New Year's resolutions, gumption has to kick in as enthusiasm wanes in mid-January.

If you set out to repair a motorcycle or assemble a metal shed (foreshadowing!) it's great to have enthusiasm — not to mention adequate light, proper tools, and helpful friends. But when none of these are available, gumption will get you past the temptation to quit.

Enthusiasm can even indicate a lack of gumption. We often drink, eat, shout our opinions, and generally act the fool with great enthusiasm, but without courage or common sense.

What else isn't gumption?

Willpower is not gumption. Willpower fails when you need it most. Willpower is simply distilled enthusiasm. It may be stronger and last longer, but willpower is still enthusiasm-based. Enthusiasm is an emotion, and your emotions are outside of your control.

The obese woman may wish with all her heart to get to a healthy weight. But how will she work through the weeks, months, and years of sensible eating and exercise after her willpower evaporates like fog over Phoenix?

Willpower is not always productive, either. The workaholic requires great willpower to grind out eighty-hour workweeks. The obsessive body builder requires great willpower to lift the weight and consume the supplements needed to have twenty-three-inch biceps. It requires great willpower to do what it takes to look mid-twentyish when you are late-fortyish. Willpower is not common sense.

What else isn't gumption?

Necessity is not gumption. It is said that Caesar burned his boats on the beaches of Kent during the invasion of Britain. That would be creating a necessity to call forth courage. Caesar's legions did indeed conquer Britain, at least enough of it to build new boats.

People with common sense don't burn their boats. They

realize they may have landed in the wrong place, that getting killed by the Britons for lack of Plan B won't help the empire.

There is another problem with relying on necessity to produce courage: the danger is often not as vivid as burning boats. Sometimes the smoke and the fire — the ill-health, divorce, bankruptcy, driving bans, and other disasters — are so far down the road that we are fooled by the illusion that there will always be time to avoid them.

Our obese friend knows she must lose weight. Chronic procrastinators know they sabotage themselves. Smokers know they must put down their cigarettes. But the disasters they face are in the future. People set off on the march to safety, but necessity generates insufficient force to keep them moving forward. They retreat. Necessity is not gumption.

What else isn't gumption?

Genius is not gumption. Genius is an endowment. A few people are born with it. Some fraction of those people find themselves in a family or field where their genius is recognizable and applicable.

The rest of us can be inspired by the likes of Shakespeare, Ben Franklin, Mozart, Einstein, Dr. King, Michael Jordan, Mother Teresa, Paul McCartney, Oprah Winfrey, and others. We may learn something from observing aspects of their behavior, but we ought not to compare ourselves to them. Their colossal accomplishments are due to a unique combination of inherited genes, phenomenal luck and superhuman appetite for hard work. This is amazing, but it is not gumption.

As the Earl of Lytton once wrote: "Genius does what it must and talent does what it can."

Mark Twain tells us to forget the idea that "Ben Franklin acquired his great genius by working for nothing, studying by moonlight, and getting up in the night instead of waiting 'til morning...these execrable eccentricities of instinct and conduct are only the *evidences* of genius, not the creators of it."

Genius, by the way, is usually not transferable outside its field.

- Michael Jordan retired from basketball and joined minor league baseball's Birmingham Barons. He had a poor batting average (and low on-base percentage) in his one season. He returned to basketball and won three more NBA championships.
- Linus Pauling won the 1954 Nobel Prize in Chemistry. He won the Nobel Peace Prize in 1962. In the 1970's he advocated loudly for vitamin C as a cure for colds, flu, and even cancer. He wrote a bestselling book on the subject. In the words of physician Paul Offit, Linus Pauling was "a man who was so spectacularly right that he won two Nobel Prizes and so spectacularly wrong that he was arguably the world's greatest quack." But still a genius.
- Sir Isaac Newton lost a fortune speculating on stock in the South Sea Company.
- Elvis.

Genius is not gumption.

How will you build your gumption? How will you make better decisions? In the sections ahead, we will examine how to be more courageous, resourceful, and how to have more common sense. First, though, let's get more facts about you.

GUMPTIONWORK

An Inquiry into
Your Goals in Life

You can do this better online:
www.gumptionade.com/inquiry-into-goals

Think of three things you want to do (lose weight, get organized, get out of debt, learn a foreign language, be a better parent, get married, play the guitar, make new friends, etc.). Use the notes section below, if you like, to come up with the three things. Take your time.

Notes

_____

_____

_____

_____

_____

_____

_____

_____

_____

_____

_____

_____

GUMPTIONWORK

Write the three things down here:

First of all, I really want to_____

_____

Second, I really want to_____

_____

I also really want to _____

_____

Transfer your answers into the spaces below. Then fill in the space after "but I cannot because." Then check the appropriate box after each sentence:

First of all, I really want to_____ ,

but I cannot because_____ .
　　This ☐ is ☐ is not largely within my personal control.

Second, I really want to_____ ,

but I cannot because_____ .
　　This ☐ is ☐ is not largely within my personal control.

I also really want to _____ ,

but I cannot because_____ .
　　This ☐ is ☐ is not largely within my personal control.

Are any of the three things that you want to do but cannot largely within your control? If yes, you either *don't* really want to do them or a powerful force is blocking you. (It must be powerful. These are the three *top things* you want to do!) More on that ahead.

GUMPTION

FUNDAMENTALS
of GUMPTION

1. People with gumption do what needs to be done, when it needs to be done, whether or not they feel like it.
2. People with gumption think and act with courage, resourcefulness, and common sense.
3. Courage is characterized by knowing, daring, and fortitude.
4. Resourcefulness is characterized by vision, creativity, and WhoHowness.
5. Common sense is characterized by logic, prudence, and curiosity.
6. Gumption may produce enthusiasm, but enthusiasm is not gumption.
7. Gumption may produce willpower, but willpower is not gumption.
8. Genius is inspiring, but it is not gumption.

II

HOW TO BE
COURAGEOUS

Chapter 6

KNOW WHAT
COURAGE IS FOR

"Everybody has a plan, until they
get punched in the mouth."

MIKE TYSON, BOXER

YOU DECIDE TO GET TO A BETTER PLACE, A
place where you will be more than you are now. You
have a new plan and new stuff. There's a new you waiting just down the road. You're *so* passionate. Finally, you're on
the right path.

Day One of the journey is fun. A warm sun beams down
out of a blue sky, flowers perfume the air, the birds sing, and
there's a spring in your step. It's all smiles to the people you
meet on the road to self-improvement. This will be shooting
fish in a barrel.

On Day Two, the fish in the barrel begin to shoot back.
There's a chill in the air. The flowers are drooping and it looks
like rain. You walk on, though, still pretty chipper: You're
gonna do this!

On Day Three, the songbirds have given way to crows, your feet are sore, and you have a headache. You keep moving, though not as far as yesterday.

On Day Four you wake up in a dark and swampy place. Your diet book is in tatters, your new running shoes are filthy, your backpack smells like garbage, and you are nauseated and depressed.

The path is now watery mud festooned with litter, poison ivy, and abandoned tires. The crows have given way to flying monkeys and your fellow travelers look like zombies.

You approach a wobbly rope bridge slung above a deep canyon. This is the border between where you are and where you want to go — between dependence and freedom. You can't recall your Day One enthusiasm.

Looking back, you spot a friendly face. Your bad habit is waving to you from a limo. It has hot coffee, blankets, dry clothes, and a light. There's a cooler in the trunk.

You realize how unpleasant your life is without your bad habit. It takes your mind off your troubles. You two share pleasing rituals: the fire ceremony of lighting a cigarette, the sacred offering of the platinum card, sexual euphoria, fragrant incense from the barbeque pit, the whirling trance of chasing the big deal, ice cubes ringing in your drink like the bells of a mountain shrine.

On Day Four you experience the real meaning of passion: suffering. How much suffering depends on how much discomfort your bad habit helps you avoid. Day Four lasts a month.

You set out on Day One to be free of your bad habit, to become better. But you need what you need right now. You

COURAGE IS FOR DEALING WITH SNAKES

A Molly Ivins story about what surprise can do to courage: Two brothers were climbing in the family hen house when they came face-to-face with a large chicken snake. They were both injured breaking down the door as they ran away.

Their mother later reminded them that chicken snakes don't hurt people. The youngest replied: "Yes Ma'am, but there are some things'll scare you so bad you hurt yourself."

Got snakes in your henhouse? Harmless things that scare you so bad you hurt yourself? That's what courage is for.

want to choose better, but you don't want to give up what you have so long enjoyed.

Courage is for confronting these two irreconcilable desires — and doing what needs to be done.

On Day Four, we retreat from the emotional strain of being responsible for ourselves. We retreat from active to passive. We retreat to our bad habit, our status quo, what doesn't require any effort. Becoming better is hard, and we are soft.

We speak of lacking willpower. What we lack is the courage to bear the suffering that comes with personal change and growth. Can we be afraid of the right things? Can we ever move on from what is comfortable?

Many people never get past Day Four. Many people never cross the border. Many people never grow up.

Unexplored places on the early maps of the world were noted with dragons and the words "There be monsters." Courage is for going *there*.

At *their roots, bad habits* are more similar than different. They are made from passive, avoidant behavior. The opposite of courage.

If your bad habit is overeating, for example, it takes courage to get to a healthy weight, and it takes courage to stay there. You have to be brave to go forward alone on Day Four, without the company of your bad habit. To bear your discomfort and see what can be done for it other than eating.

If you are obese, your body and your mind put up tremendous resistance to change. To lose weight, you have to fight:

1. Unrealistic goals that promote discouragement (What's the point? Why torture myself? I will never be thin.)
2. Shadowy but strong psychological forces

caused by the relationship between food and
feelings

3. Suspension of disbelief ("Raspberry Ketone:
Fat-Burner in a Bottle!")

4. Temptation

5. Human evolution (because Your Hairy
Ancestor had to survive famine, your body
responds to calorie reduction by increasing
metabolic efficiency — you burn fewer calories
today to do the same thing you did yesterday)

Whatever your bad habit, you have to show up for the fight
every day if you are going to make lasting change. That's what
courage is for.

On his way to Damascus, Saul of Tarsus was knocked off
his horse and temporarily blinded by a flash of light. Jesus
addressed him: "Saul, why do you persecute me? I am Jesus."

Has anyone ever had a better reason to change immediately? Yet he took three years to become St. Paul. Saul of Tarsus spent a long time in the desert, in the borderland between
Pharisee and Apostle. He was building his courage.

Will you be faster than Paul? Real change requires suffering and it requires time. Real change requires experiencing
discomfort. How much will depend on how much legitimate
suffering your bad habit has helped you avoid. That's what
courage is for.

You may also suffer from other peoples' discomfort.

Pope Urban VIII persecuted Galileo Galilei because the earth revolved around the sun.

This pope and all the popes before him accepted the conventional wisdom that the earth was at the center of the cosmos. There had been previous challenges—from Copernicus, Tycho Brahe, Bruno Giordano—but Galileo's calculations carried great weight. He campaigned for his beliefs despite having been ordered by the Church not to publicly profess the ideas of "Copernicanism."

Galileo's new fact threatened the status quo: papal infallibility and the wealth and power it supported. His Holiness had a keen interest in maintaining the status quo. If the Church was wrong about this, what else could it be wrong about?

Pope Urban had Galileo arrested to avoid recognizing a fact so threatening to Church doctrine. It took three hundred and fifty years for the Church to admit that Galileo had been correct. Given that the Church is about two thousand years old, that's equivalent to about fourteen years in the life of one person. Maybe you will be faster to admit your mistakes. I wasn't.

You too have a governing system. The status quo will resist your attempts at change, your work to become more than you are now. You too will be persecuted.

"The earth revolves around the sun," "germs cause disease," "all men are created equal" were new facts at one time. As you start to become more than you are, new facts will arise that create disorder and discomfort in your life. If your status quo includes dependence on something, you will have a fundamental resistance to independent behavior toward that thing. The fish in the barrel shoot back. That's what courage is for.

I never intended to run my own going out of business sale. As I was shutting down my advertising agency, however, my landlord demanded I clear out of his space (just because I had stopped paying rent!). I had no place to put the fifty leftover desks, chairs, computers, printers, filing cabinets, and wastebaskets. I also needed cash.

I called a secondhand office equipment dealer. He allowed that he could cart my property away for no charge. Best offer. I guess he thought I was desperate or stupid. I had just gotten over desperate. (Still working on stupid.)

I decided to sell the goods myself, piece by piece. I would have to advertise the closing of my business. I would have to advertise my failure. How humiliating. What would people think? (Turns out people don't think about me much at all, except the few who love me or hate me. None of them changed their minds because I failed at running an advertising agency.)

So I was brave and ran a three-week-long yard sale out of my eighth floor downtown office. Strictly forbidden by the terms of my lease. Put up ads in the elevators of nearby office towers. Put up more when building managers took them down. Feigned surprise and confusion when they called me to complain. Haggled, cajoled, and laughed with my customers. Sold everything down to the last three-ring binder (twenty cents).

It turned out to be profitable. It turned out to be therapeutic.

Courage Is for Dealing with Insults

A courageous way to deal with an insult is to grab the weapon your foe is wielding and turn it to your advantage. Cyrano de Bergerac is insulted at the theater about the size of his nose:

THE VISCOUNT: Sir, your nose is...very large!

CYRANO: Very!

THE VISCOUNT: Ha!

CYRANO: Is that all?

THE VISCOUNT: What do you mean?

CYRANO: Ah, no young man, that is not enough! You might have said, dear me, there are a thousand things...here you are:

Friendly: "It must be in your way while drinking; you ought to have a special beaker made!"

Descriptive: "It is a crag!...a peak!...a promontory!...A promontory did I say?...It is a peninsula!"

Off-hand: "Capital to hang one's hat upon!"...

Admiring: "What a sign for a perfumer's shop!"

Simple: "A monument! When is admission free?"...

Cyrano shows he is not ashamed. He makes the Viscount seem petty. And by making everyone laugh, he comes out on top.

A simple strategy. I didn't say easy. It does require courage. But if you have an unusual nose or other outward manifestation of differentness, you will get a lot of practice with insults. Make your answer sharp and funny, like Cyrano's. Make it like William Irvine's response to a fellow academic who said he was trying to decide whether Irvine was evil or merely misguided:

"Why can't I be both?"

It turned out to be fun. It turned out that I am more pleased with that ridiculous yard sale than with any of the glorious-looking things I did when the advertising business was great and I was on top of the world. My tree fell over, but I picked some apples before I walked away.

That's what courage is for.

I trust you don't mind examining my failures; perhaps you find them interesting. You may not find your own failures quite as entertaining. The more significant the failure — the more facts about you it reveals–the less you may care to examine it.

Watershed failures, such as divorce, arrest, and getting fired are especially rich in facts. And closely correlated with vigorous looking-away behaviors such as alcohol abuse. These golden facts are guarded by two fierce dragons, Regret and Shame. You have to be brave to pick those apples.

You won't get a lot of external reinforcement when you go searching for facts in the wreckage of your personal disaster. The world worships success and scorns failure.

The world sees no benefit in you paying attention to the facts behind your failure. The world prefers you buy the easy solutions it has to sell (Raspberry Ketones — Fat Burner in a Bottle!). But if you want to do what needs to be done, you will study your failure — and take away facts that give you better options moving forward. That's what courage is for.

Kusa Engine Company has decided to halt the development of a four-stroke lawn mower engine that runs on grass clippings. It is one brilliant engineer's baby, but the baby is over budget and behind schedule. Nevertheless, the engineer has no small amount of her self-esteem tied up in the project. She is sad and angry that the idiots who run the company see fit to close down this vital work and reassign her to Siberia (aka valve clearance specifications). She has failed.

If she is resilient, if she has courage, she will get over the setback without a career-damaging tantrum. She will move on to clean up the huge mess that valve clearance specifications has become — and perhaps put out some feelers for a new job.

Regret is an obstacle. As motorcycle maintenance author Robert Pirsig points out: "A mechanic who has a big ego to defend is at a terrific disadvantage."

You can't learn from failure if you can't get your ego down in front so you can see. Notice that Warren Buffett loudly accepts blame for his occasional investing failure. He's not afraid to admit that acquiring Dexter Shoes was a bad decision. Given his track record as the world's most successful investor, his burden of regret is light.

Ours is heavier. That's what courage is for.

Pirsig writes of a reservoir of good spirits, a savings account that can be tapped when psychic expenses are higher than expected. We call on this reserve to bounce back from adversity, or at least to keep putting one foot in front of the other. It's courage.

Some people became famous for heroic resilience: Beethoven—deaf; Helen Keller—deaf and blind; Bill Wilson—alcoholic; Franklin Roosevelt—infantile paralysis; Oprah Winfrey—abused in childhood. Heroic resilience includes anyone who transcends a childhood of deprivation and abuse—emotional, physical, or both—to become a productive adult. If that is you: well done.

But all of us have our challenges, and all of us need courage to grapple with them. To sweep things out from under the rug and name them. To let go of comfortable but outdated facts that hold us back (the earth is flat; you can't say that; I must please Dad).

Gumption is courage, resourcefulness and common sense. Courage is fundamental. It allows you to remain in possession of your common sense and resourcefulness when you really need them.

After you upset the status quo, the flying monkeys will be scary. Even so, you can laugh at their ridiculous haircuts. While you look around for an axe handle.

Everyone has a plan—until they get punched in the face. After that, everyone needs to hang in there. For ten rounds in a boxing match. For the weeks, months, and years to come in the life of any person trying to become better than they are now. That's what courage is for.

Courage *is* For

1. Right after you get punched in the mouth
2. Day Four
3. Snakes in the henhouse
4. Dealing with insults
5. Studying personal failure
6. Doing what needs to be done
7. Showing up every day

GUMPTIONWORK

It Takes Courage
to Admit a Mistake

You can do this better online:
www.gumptionade.com/admit-a-mistake

*I shall keep watching myself continually,
and—a most useful habit—shall review each
day. For this is what makes us wicked: that
no one of us looks back over his own life. Our
thoughts are devoted only to what we are
about to do. And yet our plans for the future
always depend on the past.*

Seneca, Letter Number 83

The goal of this work sheet is to learn from a mistake.

On [date] _____at [time] _____ ,

I made the following ☐ minor ☐major mistake:

_____

_____

_____

_____

_____

_____

_____

GUMPTIONWORK

I thought at the time it was the right thing to do because:

_____

_____

_____

_____

_____

_____

_____

Now, however, it seems to me that a more effective course of action would have been to:

_____

_____

_____

_____

Next time a situation like this comes up, I will try to do better as follows:

_____

_____

_____

_____

_____

Chapter 7

PUT EXCELLENCE
BEFORE SUCCESS

The Bhagavad Gita tells us we
have a right to our labor, but
not to the fruits of our labor.

STEVEN PRESSFIELD

C ONTEMPORARIES OF WILLIAM SHAKE-
speare rated him just on par with other notable
playwrights and poets. Fifty years after Shakespeare's death, John Dryden noted that the bard's plays were
being performed about half as often as those of Francis Beaumont and John Fletcher. Beaumont and Fletcher had become
more successful than Shakespeare, especially with *Philaster,*
or Love Lies a-Bleeding. You won't see that one on your Western Lit final.

By the end of the seventeenth century Shakespeare's excellence had shone through. He took the place he maintains
today as the greatest of all English-language poets and playwrights.

Success relates to the standards and opinions of others and is fleeting. Excellence relates to personal development and has enduring value. You may or may not *have* success, but you can *be* excellent.

If you must have success, you place your happiness outside of your control. Focusing on personal excellence, however, creates an internal center of gravity. As any tightrope walker will tell you, controlling your center of gravity builds courage.

Excellence is built by process: hard work, sound methods, and time. Success is influenced by luck. A person, a company, or a nation stumbles across a pair of seven-league boots and quickly laps the field. If I win $10 million in the lottery or Chevron finds vast oil deposits under my house, I am a great success.

Success is often the by-product of excellence, but excellence is never the by-product of success. In fact, brilliant success often produces arrogance, complacency, and mediocrity:

When was the last time you saw a Sony Walkman?

Why did Martha Stewart go away for five months in 2004?

How could General Motors, the leader in worldwide car sales for seventy-seven years, have filed for bankruptcy in 2009?

How far did Vanilla Ice fall from the day "Ice Ice Baby" became the first hip-hop song to hit the number one spot on the *Billboard* chart?

The drive for excellence is about building legitimate pride in the growing mastery of a skill — gardening, say, or swimming, playing the cello, selling shoes, or using Excel spreadsheets.

The drive for success, however, is often rooted in vanity, that is, the usually doomed attempt to feel worthy by making others see you as worthy.

Pursue excellence and you will be in control of your center of gravity. Pursue excellence and you will build your courage.

The Difference between Success and Excellence

Focused on success	Focused on excellence
The result	The performance
Failure is not an option	Failure is a teacher
The destination	The journey
Winning	Fulfilling potential
Can't stand to be beaten	Can't stand to be outworked
Opponents are a threat	Opponents make me better
Power over others	Power over myself
The end justifies the means	There's a right way and a wrong way
Building reputation	Building character

The late Joe Paterno, head football coach at Penn State University for almost fifty years, once spoke brilliantly about the meaning of excellence:

There are many people, particularly in sports, who think that success and excellence are the same thing. They are not the same thing.

Excellence is something that is lasting and dependable and largely within a person's control. In contrast, success is perishable and is often outside our control. If you strive for excellence, you will probably be successful eventually.

Remarkable words. How sad that Joe Paterno's hard-earned reputation as an excellent teacher and leader is blackened.

In 2012, Jerry Sandusky, a long-time assistant Penn State football coach, was convicted of 45 counts of molesting children, sometimes in football team facilities. The university commissioned a report on the matter by ex-FBI director Louis Freeh. He assigned significant blame to Paterno and other university officials:

The most powerful men at Penn State failed to take any steps for 14 years to protect the children who Sandusky victimized. Messrs. Spanier, Schultz, Paterno and Curley never demonstrated, through actions or words, any concern for the safety and well-being of Sandusky's victims until after Sandusky's arrest.

This is not excellence.

Joe Paterno announced his impending retirement but got fired instead. He wrote: "This is a tragedy. It is one of the great sorrows of my life. I wish I had done more."

Simple, not easy. The Jerry Sandusky scandal is a lesson in the difficulty of putting excellence before success. As is the steady stream of hypocrisy and misbehavior flowing from other college football programs across the country.

Let's follow the money. Successful major college football programs are gushers of prestige, power, and cash. Penn State risked losing some of each by reporting Jerry Sandusky's crimes to the police.

This would have saved other children from sexual exploitation, but it would also have brought scandal to the football program. Player recruitment might have been hindered by bad publicity. Success on the field might have been temporarily imperiled. Contributions to the athletic program might have gone down. Television money was at risk.

The Penn State officials had a choice. They could have done the hard thing — the right thing — and invited legitimate suffering by exposing Sandusky's illegal and immoral behavior. When the big test came, however, they chose success over excellence. They failed the victims of Jerry Sandusky. They failed their players. They failed their employer. Above all, they failed themselves. The impact of the scandal was an order of magnitude greater than it would have been had they done the excellent thing and gone to the police immediately.

Remember Joe Paterno's valuable words on excellence, of course. Learn from the mistakes at Penn State, certainly. Be more courageous, if you can, when your big test comes. Simple. Not easy.

Focusing on success and results — "I have to be thin; I need to make lots of money; I must win a Pulitzer" — is less effective than aspiring to personal development — "I want to be more than I am now; I want to be the best poet I can be; I want to be sober today; I want to do my best work and get paid for it."

So I am not the sharpest knife in the drawer. I will never be Nassim Taleb, Adam Gopnick, Malcolm Gladwell, Roberto

Martinez, or Michael Lewis. What then? I can still write a good book—this book. I can still coach my son's soccer team the best I can. I can still be excellent. I can still be courageous. Marcus Aurelius put it this way:

> You will never be remarkable for quick-wittedness. Be it so.... Cultivate [what is] within your power: sincerity, for example, and dignity; industriousness, and sobriety...be frugal, considerate, and frank; be temperate in manner and in speech; carry yourself with authority. See how many qualities there are which could be yours at this moment.

It will help you be more courageous if you know about the triad of control. Everything that happens can be put in one of three buckets:

1. Things over which you have no control: the sun rising in the morning; the Supreme Court's decision on gay marriage; where the Dow Jones Industrial Average will end the day. Spend no time worrying about these.
2. Things over which you have partial control: the quality of your relationship with your spouse; the long term growth of your savings; advancement in your profession; your golf score; how your children fare in life. Do your best at creating good outcomes in these areas

but do not depend on them for your happiness.
Stuff happens.

3. Things over which you have complete control:
    how you treat your spouse and children; the
    quality of your work; what you eat; what you
    drink; whether you smoke; what you do to be
    the best golfer you can be; how hard you work
    toward any personal or professional goal, on
    or off the golf course. Think first upon these
    things and your courage will grow.

Be wary of people or products that focus on outcome
("instant weight loss") over process ("this can help you in your
work of getting to a healthy weight"). Focus on the journey
rather than the destination. There are no elevators to the top
of the mountain you are climbing.

Put excellence before success and you will build your
courage.

FUNDAMENTALS *of* EXCELLENCE

1. Success is an outcome, dependent on luck and the opinions of others.
2. Excellence is a process: hard work, sound methods, and time.
3. Excellence is under your direct control.
4. Success is fleeting, but excellence endures.
5. The pursuit of success can lead you far away from excellence.

Counting Kudos
Make Excellence Visible

You can find a blank template for your own kudos
list online at **www.gumptionade.com/kudos**

Make a record of your history of excellence in whatever
format works best for you. Here are excerpts from your
author's "Kudos List" over a couple of years to show you one
way to do it. I built the list by recording examples of personal
excellence, large and small. I read it every once in a while to
remind myself.

Scale:
☆ Excellence is small but noteworthy
☆ Excellence is medium
☆ A large chunk o' excellence
☆ **Jumbo excellence**

2014
☆ Remembered to not eat breakfast and get to doctor's
office on time for lab work.
☆ Went to 3-hour evening seminar with D, because she
wanted to.
☆ Remembered to notice D's new hairstyle and
compliment her on it.
☆ Got AT&T to upgrade me after Internet
connection went down.
☆ Changed password on my bank account.
☆ Made dinner *and* cleaned it up for tired wife.
☆ Walked to grocery store for exercise, got fresh tomatoes
for dinner.
☆ Finished *Gumptionade* Draft #7.
☆ Sat through awful foodie movie with D.

GUMPTIONWORK

☆ Attended the Outreach meeting after church.

☆ Heavy weights workout at the Y.

☆ Called B just to say hello.

☆ Kept my working discipline and did not read emails constantly all day.

☆ Picked up T from rehab so she could go to the church dinner.

☆ Got a jump on finding a copy editor today, a few weeks before I will need one.

☆ Filed Pastoral Care team report on time.

☆ Fixed the new business proposal immediately after getting request for changes.

☆ Resisted binge-watching *Orange Is the New Black*, so I could get up early and write.

☆ Swam 45 minutes at the Y when I really didn't feel like it.

☆ Called sister on her birthday.

☆ 40 minutes of exercise on the elliptical in hot attic.

☆ Did not eat any of the cupcakes served after church.

☆ Figured out how to stream shows from Netflix onto the TV.

☆ 401k deposit made on time.

☆ Sent out client billing for July on August 1!

☆ Wrapped D's birthday presents the night before, so they would be on the breakfast table when she woke up.

☆ Turned off the TV and went to bed at a decent hour so I could be up early to write.

☆ Programmed new garage door remote.

☆ Remembered to do change of address at bank (had to be done in person) when I deposited a check.

☆ Researched two Network Solutions charges on my Amex bill, found out they were not something I ordered, and got the promise of a full refund – over $100!

☆ Birthday gift for sister.

☆ Was patient, did not jump on B for not making appointment with F, and it turned out not really to be B's fault.

☆ I salute you for getting this far in my kudos list!

☆ Picked up veggies for tonight's dinner on the way back from the bank.

☆ Swam for 45 minutes after work.

GUMPTIONWORK

☆ Completed project for FM: doing what you said you would do, when you said you would do it, despite unforeseen difficulties.

☆ K, M and E comments on *Gumptionade* draft #5 reviewed and followed-up on.

☆ Pastoral care visits made on the way home from church.

☆ Battery, tires and oil change for the Corolla.

☆ N says *Gumptionade* is "ready to go" to press.

☆ Made that uncomfortable call to Smith, re: Payne.

☆ Gift sent to S: gratitude expressed promptly.

2013

☆ 300 + workouts in 2013.

☆ Good meeting with J.

☆ Gumptionade draft #5 off to M.

☆ Good meetings with J and P.

☆ G to ER in Bridgeport in the middle of the night.

☆ Mounted guitar on wall of office.

☆ 4 letters to Uncle G in October.

☆ Kicked off Ireland trip planning.

☆ Project follow up, to show S and T that I do what I say I will do.

☆ M&A call with Consultant.

☆ Practicing with online meeting product.

☆ Drove L to the municipal lot—in the middle of the workday—so she could reclaim her car that was towed.

☆ If you are *still* reading my kudos list, go to www.gumptionade.com/dream-reader and claim a prize.

☆ Sf.com work for client – taking my capabilities up a notch.

☆ Amex green card: miles transferred off, card closed.

☆ SodaStream® refill. What a pain. First world problem.

☆ Patience with D, with myself.

☆ Remembered wedding anniversary and did something about it.

☆ January mileage done in January.

☆ Eight days in a row of waiting until 4 PM before checking my Facebook feed.

GUMPTIONWORK

Start your own kudos list.

You can find a blank template for your own kudos list online at **www.gumptionade.com/kudos**

> **Scale:**
> ☆ Excellence is small but noteworthy
> ☆ Excellence is medium
> ☆ A large chunk o' excellence
> ☆ **Jumbo excellence**

_____

_____

_____

_____

_____

_____

_____

_____

_____

_____

_____

_____

_____

_____

Chapter 8

TRANSLATE UNCERTAINTY INTO RISK

Should I stay or should I go?

THE CLASH

I T IS LIKELY THAT THE MERCHANT SHIP *Wigan Thistle* will get to Stockholm to deliver its load of British goods. It is likely that the ship will then return to London with Swedish timber, hemp, and bar iron. But its owner Francis McKnight is worried—if it does not, he will be ruined.

This is the early 18th century. Bad weather, French privateers, or poor navigation could result in a total loss and debtors' prison for McKnight. The *Wigan Thistle* is his livelihood. He has to put his ship to sea, but he can't bear the risk of losing it.

Deciding how best to proceed under conditions of uncertainty is a fundamental problem of living. The solution is to transform uncertainty into risk when you can. Risk is a thing that can be measured. Sometimes you can pay other people to take risk from you — you can insure against it.

Francis McKnight goes to Lloyd's Coffee House on Lombard Street to buy some courage. Others are there, ready to sell it. In return for a payment now, they promise to make good on the loss McKnight might sustain from the *Wigan Thistle's* upcoming voyage.

Ben Watson takes on part of McKnight's risk. So do nine other investors present at Lloyd's that day. McKnight can now send his ship out on the North Sea. He has courage.

There is a tool for transforming uncertainty into risk. It's called statistics.

Like the other underwriters, Watson has access to tables that list voyages attempted and completed, and ships lost at sea. Watson has access to statistics. He knows his risk of coughing up one-tenth of the value of the *Wigan Thistle* and its cargo.

He will not be ruined if the ship goes down. And if it completes its voyage, as is statistically likely, his one-tenth of McKnight's risk premium is pure profit. Statistics give Watson the courage to risk a moderate loss in return for a more likely small gain.

Good business on both sides. Uncertainty was turned into risk, which could be bought and sold. This is a way to be courageous.

Let's look at another example of purchasing risk reduction — and use statistics to decide whether it's good business too.

Overweight twenty-first-century American Joe Hart reads that men with high cholesterol are fifty percent more likely to have a heart attack in the next ten years than other men their age. This news makes Joe uncertain. He has high cholesterol.

Joe attempts to lower his risk. He gets a prescription for a drug to decrease the cholesterol in his blood. It comes with side effects — headaches, muscle weakness, and a one thousand-dollar per year out of pocket cost. The discomfort seems worthwhile. After all, he *is* cutting his risk of heart attack a lot.

Would Joe change his mind if he looked at the facts behind that apparently large risk reduction? Here are the statistics:

- Four out of one hundred men his age *without* elevated cholesterol are expected to have a heart attack in the next ten years.
- The number is six out of one hundred for men his age *with* elevated cholesterol.

That alarming fifty percent increase in heart attack risk is a matter of two more heart attacks per one hundred men. Over ten years. Even if they *don't* take that drug, ninety-four out of one hundred men *with* elevated cholesterol will *not* have a heart attack in the next ten years.

The fifty percent figure is a measure of *relative frequency*. Figures that cite numbers — e.g., from four to six heart attacks per one hundred men — are measures of *actual frequency*. Insist upon actual frequency when you weigh risk.

Joe may decide that the difference between four and six does not merit the side effects of the drug. Trying to eliminate every risk from life is neither courageous nor possible. Translating his uncertainty into his risk of a coronary gives Joe the courage to do what needs to be done about his heart. He may choose wrong, but he will not be guessing.

There is much uncertainty among twenty-first-century Americans about breast cancer, prostate cancer, and cardiovascular disease, to name a few threats to our health. Some risks are exaggerated; others are ignored. Most of us aren't doing what needs to be done about our health.

Similarly, there is great uncertainty about risk in the stock market, as we learned during the crash of 2008. Most of us aren't doing what needs to be done about our money.

We pay too little attention to what is actually dangerous, and too much to what is actually not.

> *Statistical thinking will one day be as necessary for efficient citizenship as the ability to read and write.*
> H. G. WELLS

You live in an uncertain world. You may have a fine day tomorrow, or you may get a pie in the face. A lot of clowns out there. You just don't know.

You have to make decisions, regardless. You have to make decisions under conditions of uncertainty:

- Is he the one for me?
- What is the best car in my price range?
- Should we launch in this weather?

- Is it time to sell?
- Should I have that operation?
- Can this wait?
- How high can I put my deductible?

It is important to translate uncertainty into risk. It is just as important to translate *certainty* into risk. This reduces your chance of acting on optimism, such as: "I will change him." Or "this will only take a week." Or "safe as houses."

By measuring risk, statistics defend you against your own recklessness and the recklessness of others. Go Fever is not courageous. Neither is avoiding all risk.

Because risk can be weighed, it can be priced. There are markets for buying and selling risk, such as the coffee shop that became Lloyd's of London. There are times you want to buy down your risk, like Francis McKnight. There are times you may not, as Joe Hart saw.

What are *you* risking? Don't guess. Know.

Go Fever won't get you through Day Four. It takes courage to become more than you are now. Effective risk evaluation builds courage. Unfortunately, it *requires two things that are in short supply among most humans:*

1. the ability to monitor the effect of emotions on judgment, and
2. the ability to use statistics as a tool.

The human brain is millions of years older than statistics. Statistical thinking was not a deciding factor in how Your Hairy Ancestor made her prehistoric living on the African savannah. It was not passed down to you by natural selection or provided by an intelligent design. Neither was statistical thinking gifted to you by your other ancestor, The Child You Were. In the earliest years in your personal evolution, you weren't ready for 2 + 2.

You are almost certainly now, as I was before I wrote this chapter, innumerate when it comes to the math needed to effectively evaluate risk. Few modern humans, including few doctors, professors, and CEOs, have the required grasp of basic statistics.

Do you judge tornadoes to be more risky than asthma? You are about twenty times more likely to be killed by asthma. People believe otherwise because tornadoes are more vivid.

If you've ever seen them in person, you know how terrifying tornadoes are. They even make a dramatic impression on video. Asthma? Not so much.

Speaking of asthma: A friend of mine accepts the risk of smoking, which costs women an average of 4.6 years of life. She will not, however, accept the risk of living near a nuclear power plant, less dangerous than riding a bicycle. But stories about nuclear power plant disasters are easy to remember.

People are afraid of the wrong things. They judge they are more likely to die in an accident than by disease. They think they are more likely to be murdered than to commit suicide. Statistics show that disease causes about sixteen times as many deaths as accidents, and suicide occurs twice as frequently as murder. Accidents and murders are simply more interesting and more widely reported.

Buy a gun if it makes you feel safer, but know that — statistically — you are more likely to shoot yourself than someone trying to do you harm.

People believe otherwise because we tend to assess risk based on emotion — how much we fear something — rather than how dangerous it really is. People judge risk by the ease with which examples come to mind and how vivid those examples are.

One reason lottery tickets sell so well to innumerate people is that they make great wealth quite easy to imagine. You are about one hundred times more likely to be killed by lightning than you are to win a million-dollar lottery prize. Perhaps you still want to buy that ticket. At least you are not guessing. You have statistics.

The weakness in human risk evaluation is the stock-in-trade of terrorists. They do flashy, horrible things to a minuscule subset of the population and thereby attempt to intimidate the rest. It is not courageous to respond by crying for more government protection, surrendering our civil rights, or lashing out. Effective risk evaluation is key to responding effectively — courageously — to terrorists. Simple. Not easy.

Experts are not immune to misjudging risk. Many American physicians unknowingly overstate the risk of prostate and breast cancer while also understating the risk of treatment.

Former chairman of the Federal Reserve Alan Greenspan was shocked when the housing bubble burst, causing a worldwide economic recession. He says now that he "made a mistake in presuming" that the giant financial firms would regulate themselves. That was naive, but it was not Greenspan's worst mistake. His worst mistake was ignoring the existential risk to the U.S. economy if the giant financial firms did *not* regulate themselves, regardless of his presumptions. *Optimism is not courage.*

Levee failures caused 80 percent of New Orleans to flood during Hurricane Katrina. 1,833 people died. The American Society of Civil Engineers noted afterward that Louisiana officials did not account for "...the probability of failure combined with the consequences to human health and safety if that failure were to occur." Like Greenspan, Louisiana officials presumed that low risk of a catastrophic event meant they did not need to prepare for it. *Voluntary myopia is not courage.*

Perhaps the most damning finding of the investigation into the *Challenger* space shuttle disaster concerned the misstating of risk. NASA management put forward a 1 in 100,000 chance of catastrophic failure. Their own engineers felt the chances were closer to 1 in 200. NASA management embraced the illusion of certainty. *Go Fever is not courage.*

Consider other examples of how we misjudge risk:

1. The rate of deaths from skydiving accidents remains stable despite great advances in equipment safety. Emboldened skydivers try riskier dives.
2. Helmets are the main reason there are so many head injuries in football.
3. Otherwise sane adults make phone calls while driving.

Tom is a turkey. He lives on a farm. Farmer brings him delicious corn to eat and fresh, cool water to drink every day.

The pattern repeats faithfully for 1,000 days. Using inductive reasoning — deriving a general principle from specific observations — Tom becomes certain that Farmer is a benevolent creature that exists to meet his needs.

Tom does wonder, sometimes: "Farmer takes milk from the cow and apples from the tree. Why would he give me everything I need and expect nothing in return?" Or "what became of that older turkey that disappeared last year? Or the one before that?"

When the gate is left open, Tom does not muster the courage to escape into the woods. Why would he? The woods seem uncomfortable. The farm is comfortable.

Perhaps it will remain so. Or perhaps Tom is a Magoo.

On day 1,001, Tom's fate manifests itself, ax in hand. Perhaps Tom should have translated his uncertainty into his risk of becoming Thanksgiving dinner.

How to Avoid
Guessing about Risk

Most of us are vulnerable to the dangerous illusion called the false positive. To demonstrate, please allow me to make you sick.

You have been feeling tired for a long while and your skin is becoming painfully dry. Your doctor suspects you have Finding's Pneumonia (named for Sir Basil Finding; called FindingPneumo for short). She orders a test. It can only be given once. You test positive.

Your doctor informs you that without treatment, FindingPneumo will shortly cause your skin to turn bright orange and scaly for about three years.

There is a cure. She recommends you take it. It has side effects, however: severe flulike symptoms for two months. It costs $28,000 and is not covered by your insurance.

You are uncertain. Should you buy the cure? What is your risk? You ask for more facts. Your doctor gives you these:

1. Three percent of the population has FindingPneumo, whether or not they have symptoms yet. She unnecessarily points out—you are not an idiot—that 97 percent of the population does *not* have FindingPneumo.

2. The test for FindingPneumo is
not perfectly accurate. There is a
10 percent chance of a false positive.
That is to say, one out of ten people
who do *not* have FindingPneumo will
nonetheless get a test result that
says they do.

3. There is also a 67 percent chance
that a person who actually *has*
FindingPneumo will test positive for
it. That leaves a 33 percent chance of
a false negative.

You seek a second opinion. That doctor tells you
exactly the same thing, as does Wikipedia.

Now you must decide. Should you spend $28,000
and feel horrible for sixty days to ensure that you do
not look like a clown fish for three years?

Yes, you did test positive, but what is the chance
it was a false positive? Do you really have Finding-
Pneumo? The test is only 67 percent accurate, after
all.

So you have a 67 percent chance of having the disease, right? Wrong.

An estimate of 57 percent, however, neatly sub-
tracts the 10 percent false positive number from
67 percent. Also wrong.

Channel your inner Gene Kranz. Be a good flight
director. Don't guess. Know. Assess your risk with

statistics. Just how strong a piece of evidence is the fact that you tested positive for Finding-Pneumo?

Imagine that Flight Director Kranz gives you this big hint: "Base rates." Imagine you ask him to elaborate and he says: "Ninety-seven percent of the population is a lot of people."

The thought then occurs to you that a large number of people must get false positives. Indeed the 10 percent false positive rate multiplied by the 97 percent of the population who don't have Find-ingPneumo means that 9.7 percent of the population will get a false positive if tested.

You see that the false positive group would be more than three times larger than the 3 percent of all people who actually *have* FindingPneumo. Feeling a bit better, you proceed to turn your uncertainty into risk. You get out pen and paper and proceed to draw the diagram opposite this page.

Now you know your risk. You have a less than one in five chance of becoming bright orange and scaly. Maybe you will keep your $28,000 and skip the side effects of the medicine. Maybe you won't. You certainly won't be guessing.

Regardless of your choice—or the result—you have done what needs to be done by someone who tests positive for FindingPneumo. That's excellent.

Does a Positive Test Mean I Have FindingPneumo?

For every 1,000 People Tested:

Group H
30 People Have
FindingPneumo
(3% of 1,000)

Group D
970 People Don't Have
FindingPneumo
(97% of 1,000)

20 Will Test
Positive
(67% of 30)

10 Will Test
Negative
(33% of 30)

97 Will Test
Positive
(10% of 970)

873 Will Test
Negative
(90% of 970)

Since I tested positive, I need to know the probability of **ANYONE** testing positive actually having the disease. To start, I will add the number of people who test positive from both groups:

20 from Group H + 97 from Group D = 117 total people who tested positive

I will turn uncertainty into risk by seeing what percentage of that 117 people who tested positive are the 20 people who test positive and actually do <u>HAVE</u> the disease:

20 ÷ 117 = 0.17

Because I tested positive, my probability of having FindingPneumo is **17%**.

In *The Black Swan*, Nassim Taleb uses the turkey problem to point out that recent history is not conclusive. Safety is in effective risk assessment. Unlikely-but-catastrophic scenarios must be addressed. Tomorrow is one day closer to day 1,001. Courage is in more and better facts. Courage is in statistics.

Here are a few statistics everyone should know:

1. Smoking increases the risk of coronary heart disease and stroke by two to four hundred percent and lung cancer by over two thousand percent.
2. Approximately five percent of the general adult population has a sex addiction.
3. Women who identified their work as highly stressful were forty percent more likely to suffer from heart disease than female colleagues reporting lower work-related stress.
4. Individual investors who trade actively reduce their returns by about four percent annually versus investors who buy and hold low-cost mutual funds.
5. Obesity increases the risk of:
    *   diabetes by seven hundred percent,
    *   heart disease by eighty-one percent,
    *   stroke by sixty-four percent,
    *   depression by fifty-five percent,

- asthma by fifty percent,
- Alzheimer's by forty-two percent, and
- getting ten types of cancer.

6. Twenty-five percent of women who have more than seven alcoholic drinks per week are considered to be dependent on alcohol.

People with gumption look for facts and options. They also know the difference between paying attention and useless worrying. They don't gamble more than they can afford to lose, but they do accept the risks inherent in living a purposeful, adult life. That requires courage — and statistics.

Some of your certainty about who you are and what you can do is no better than a guess. You can do more. Start with your understanding of risk and probabilities. You accept too much risk in some areas (e.g., your bad habits) and too little in others. You take advice from people who are themselves just guessing.

It's a good thing to be literate: You can read food labels, you can read Shakespeare, and you can read the funnies. But if you want to be courageous — neither cowardly nor rash — it pays to be numerate. Look at the statistics. Measure real risk. There be dragons. There be courage. There be gumption.

FUNDAMENTALS
of TRANSLATING
UNCERTAINTY into RISK

1. Do not confuse what is frightening with what is dangerous.

2. Do not confuse what you want to happen with what is likely to happen.

3. Use available statistics to measure your uncertainty before making big decisions.

4. Use actual frequency not relative frequency (that fifty percent increase may only be from four to six out of one hundred).

5. Accept the risks inherent in living a purposeful, adult life.

6. Insure yourself against potentially ruinous losses.

7. Don't insure your microwave oven.

8. Certainty is an illusion: beware the false positive.

9. Things often seem more orderly than they are — one-hundred-year floods can happen twice in two years.

10. Most smart people are not smart about statistics.

Look, Ma —
Watch Me Measure
Uncertainty!

You can do this better online:
www.gumptionade.com/measure-uncertainty

I now place two dice on a table in front of you. They appear identical, but one is fixed to land only on three or six. I then offer to bet you ten dollars that you can't guess which of the dice is fixed, after rolling just one.

You take the bet. Hey, it's just ten bucks. You pick one up and roll it. It lands on six. This is almost certainly the fixed dice. That was easy.

Before you can say anything, though, I offer to up the bet to one thousand dollars.

You are pretty sure that would be a good bet for you, but...a grand? You are uncertain. At this point you cannot afford to guess. Before you make the big bet, you need to weigh your risk of losing one thousand dollars.

Can you can use logic to translate your uncertainty into risk? If you hated FindingPneumo, think of this exercise as preparation for Chapter 9: "Suffer Better." Please proceed:

Since it came up six, the probability I rolled the fixed dice is as follows:

_____

You aren't sure? Look at it this way:

GUMPTIONWORK

Bayesian Probability Analysis

	FIXED DICE	FAIR DICE
Probability you chose each dice	1 in 2 (=½)	1 in 2 (=½)
Probability of rolling a "6" with it	1 in 2 (=½)	1 in 6 (=⅙)
Combining the probabilities	½ x ½ (= **¼**)	½ x ⅙ (=**1/12**)

One-quarter is three times larger than one-twelfth. Because you rolled a six, you are three times more likely to have picked the fixed dice than the fair dice. This is the same as saying there is a seventy-five percent chance you picked the fixed dice.

You are no longer uncertain. If you bet that the dice you rolled is the fixed one, your risk of losing is twenty-five percent. Take the bet if you can afford to buy a seventy-five percent chance of winning one thousand dollars, accompanied by a twenty-five percent chance of losing that much.

Extra credit: Show yourself why this $1,000 bet is worth $500:

_____

_____

_____

_____

_____

_____

Chapter 9

SUFFER BETTER

Where is it written that you're
supposed to be happy all the time?

Sylvia Boorstein

I
F YOU WANT TO AVOID SUFFERING, DON'T
build a metal storage shed from a kit you buy at Lowe's.
I did, to please my ex-wife during the final stretch of our
doomed marriage. We needed more storage space because the
garage was filled with cats she had rescued.

When I say "metal storage shed from a kit," what I mean is
this: hundreds of wobbly sheet metal pieces with sharp edges
and spear-tip corners, several large bags of pointy screws and
plastic doodads, and a 2×3-foot sheet of inscrutable instruc-
tions, folded up like a road map. Floor not included (appar-
ent only after work has begun).

I am not handy. I respond poorly to directions, written or
verbal. Words cannot convey how much I hated that kit from
the moment I opened the four hundred pound box. And how
much it hated me back.

Any enthusiasm I might have had for the work was swamped by the oppressive August-in-Memphis heat and humidity, mosquito clouds, a work site fouled by a constantly renewed supply of turds from my ex-wife's dogs (no doubt intended as encouragement), and my ridiculous tool kit (a hammer, a Phillips head screwdriver, a broken steak knife).

I promised I would build the metal shed before I understood what that meant. Now I had to. I needed proof that I was a person who did what he said he would do, even if it sucked a thousand times more than he could have imagined. Which it did. Even if the process caused him great suffering. Which it certainly did.

Worked it every day, rain or shine. Started over five times. Made fundamental mistakes at every important juncture. Cut myself, stabbed myself, dropped heavy things on my toes, and cursed like a sailor. Finished in October. Angry throughout.

I thought I was angry because I had allowed my ex-wife to persuade me that this Rubik's Cube with a roof was better than a prebuilt wooden shed, that *any* storage shed was better than just clearing that tribe of cats out of the garage. I thought I was angry that this marriage was failing, that my first marriage failed, that my business was failing.

Sometime after metal shed Day Four, however, I realized what I was really angry about — my own complicity in all the problems heaped upon me, symbolized so perfectly by this absurd project.

Here's the not-absurd thing, though. I had been retreating for years, but when I got to the metal shed, I turned and fought. I wrestled with that bad boy for six weeks and got it built. There were no pieces left over at the end. I threw them away.

I wanted self-respect, not vengeance. Passion gave me the courage to persevere at something more than what I thought I could accomplish. Suffering through the building of that metal shed made me better than I was.

Sometime after Day Four I could see a new fact: To avoid pointless suffering in the future I had to stop being so impulsive, so passive, so eager to please. I had to stop automatically going along with other people's agendas and then being angry about it. I had to start thinking things through on the front end. I had to act more like a grown-up.

The metal shed stood for two weeks. Then a mighty wind came and flattened it with a tree. A petulant leave-taking by the forces of chaos, self-loathing, and inertia I had just defeated. It only increased my sense of triumph. Take the metal shed. I'll keep the new fact.

Peter Habeler has climbed five of the fourteen 8,000+ meter mountains of the world. He and Reinhold Messner were the first to reach the summit of the tallest, Mount Everest, without supplemental oxygen. The ascent required weeks of preparation and days of intense physical and mental exertion.

Habeler has a passion for climbing mountains. During the Everest ascent, he suffered from cold, hunger, thirst, fatigue, blisters, cramps, and oxygen deprivation. But his view from the summit — the roof of the world — was spectacular.

What if, instead of making the climb, he had watched a brilliant IMAX documentary about scaling Everest and then been whisked to the summit by special helicopter? You know what. Entertainment is not achievement.

The meaning of the climb was generated by the process, not by the outcome. It came from the passion — the suffering — required to get there and back. The tougher things got, the more meaningful it was to keep putting one foot in front of the other.

What if a whiteout blizzard made further progress impossible after Habeler reached the Hillary Steps, three hundred feet below the summit? Recall the triad of control: the weather on Mount Everest is one of the things over which Habeler has no control. I think he would have been disappointed in the result, but satisfied with his own performance. His part was hard, and he did his part.

Habeler's Everest journey was suffering in service of a higher goal, a goal he set for himself in cooperation with Reinhold Messner and a formidable mountain in Tibet. His suffering created meaning. It created achievement. It created courage.

Suffering over things you cannot control is normal, but it is not creative. It builds anxiety, it builds frustration, but it does not build courage.

You want more money, sure, but try not to be passionate about the stock market. Your suffering will be pointless. Unless you are the Chair of the Federal Reserve, the stock market is one of the things over which you have no control.

Make yourself sit down and write a budget instead, as a first step toward increasing your financial security. Creative suffering — creating a comfortable retirement — will mean driving your serviceable car another few years instead of buying that twin-turbo status symbol you covet. If you're one of those people whose self-esteem is bound up with the car they drive, your ego will contract painfully as your savings grow. This is suffering for a purpose. This is creative.

Your passion will give you the courage to stand fast against the rampant consumerism of your brother-in-law, who drives over on Thanksgiving in the BMW 328i you once wanted. He can't afford it either. And he gets it in white, which is ridiculous.

Do you suffer when people wrong you? Do you inflict more suffering on yourself by carrying a grudge over it? Normal, but not creative. By relinquishing your equanimity, you pile insult on top of the injury you have already sustained. You suffer without meaning.

Suffer better: try to understand what might have caused your friend to let you down, why your spouse nags you, what makes your boss so irritable, your teenager so contrary. Under what circumstances might you do the same? Make your suffering creative: try to understand and forgive the person. Look for your part in this.

Not to say you should accept mistreatment. Not to say that you shouldn't stay away from out-of-control people. Move on from the abuser. Let that demented driver who flips you the bird zoom out of sight and out of mind. He has nothing to teach you.

To paraphrase Carl Jung, your bad habit is always a substitute for creative suffering. Naturally, then, it is only through creative suffering that it can be supplanted.

How can you tell if your suffering is creative? Well, does it make you more courageous, or less? Creative suffering increases fortitude.

American writer Paul Theroux wrote about a break up with a woman: "The memory of pain can itself be a pain-killer."

Like many others, for a time my beloved father chose to drink vodka as a way to lessen the pain of living. That was not creative. Creative suffering is to turn and fight: Experience the pain and search out the cause. Ask for help. So simple to talk about. So hard to do. His injuries were great. Your injuries may be great.

If you continue to drink vodka as a way to lessen the pain of living, you are still going to suffer, of course. But your suffering will be pointless: hangovers; lost wallets; lost weekends; DWIs; unemployment; liver disease. A better alternative: suffer to become more than you are now. Suffer better.

There are no shortcuts to a healthy weight, healthy relationships, financial security, sobriety or self-respect. You add meaning by the work you put in along the way. Without meaning, you cannot bear the discomfort involved in becoming more than you are now. Without meaning there is not enough courage to keep walking on Day Four.

There are no helicopter rides to personal growth. Because there is money to be made, however, many people try to sell you a ticket.

In the glory days of the British navy, sailors were punished by flogging. It didn't make them better. If Jack Tar chose not to curse Bill Bobstay again, it wasn't because he had changed his mind about the bosun. Jack simply didn't want another dozen. By taking his punishment, Jack paid his debt to the ship. If he survived, he recovered his full duties and privileges.

There is a difference between punishment and sacrifice. Punishment is suffering that breeds resentment, resistance, and ultimately rebellion. It's not creative.

If you consider your attempts at self-improvement to be punishment, why would you continue to suffer on Day Four? You've been tied to the whipping post. You've earned the right to resume your privileges — your bad habit.

Sacrifice is also suffering — it hurts to grow. It's painful to force yourself to get out of bed an hour early to run or do yoga or study. To avoid foods you crave. To listen to what you don't want to hear. To change dead-end routines. But if you accept this suffering out of self-respect, it's not punishment. It's a choice. Your choice. You make a sacrifice to the person you will be tomorrow.

So many self-improvement projects fail on Day Four because they feel like punishment, something that is happening *to* you. Flogging will not improve morale. Punishment does not originate from self-respect. It will not build self-discipline. It will not build courage. Suffer better.

Preparation stores courage like a battery stores electricity. Preparation is creative suffering that increases the courage you need to do something hard. Maybe you practice hundreds of hours in order to play a piano recital. Or you write ten drafts of a book. Or you start keeping your New Year's resolutions on December 1st.

The problem isn't that the things we want to do are too hard. The problem is that we are too soft. Preparation is suffering *now* to give you courage later. Courage to persevere, courage to face the possibility of failing. You might walk onstage, sit down at the piano, and stumble all over the first movement. Your book might be ignored. You might not lose a pound with your sensible eating. Your injured knee may never let you finish that marathon. There might be a blizzard when you get to the Hillary Steps. Preparation hardens you by building courage. You will do *your* part.

The many flight simulations carried out by Mission Control prior to the launch of *Apollo 13* were preparation. Preparation also includes repeated experiences of failure survived and learned from: failure to control drinking, by Ann Richards; failure to thrive as a professional baseball player, by Billy Beane.

Julia Hill's gospel-soaked, space-constrained childhood prepared her well for a self-imposed sentence of 738 days on two
six-foot-by-six-foot plywood platforms in a tree 180 feet closer
to heaven. She might have been eccentric, but she was not
soft. Courage.

Preparation reduces risk. Things that look dangerous are
made routine by repeated practice. You can get good at riding a motorcycle upside down in a small round cage, repairing eyeballs with a laser beam, or buying the debt of bankrupt
companies.

Preparation is creative suffering. It builds courage. Are you
preparing yourself to do better?

"Judge not lest ye be judged" is more than a New Testament
admonition. It is a call to suffer better. It is a call to be compassionate. It accounts for the most important thing psychologists know: The mistakes people make are much easier to see
than the underlying causes.

An experiment with divinity school students found that they
were significantly less likely to stop and help a person in dis-
tress if they were in a hurry to get across campus. It is possible
that the Good Samaritan was not running late to a meeting.

Why people do what they do is hard to discern. You don't
know what pressure some people are under. You don't know
what is going on in their heads, what boons or injuries they
carry around between their ears. You likely don't know what
boons or injuries you carry around between your own ears.

Compassion builds courage. A greasy, smiling man with shabby clothing and bloodshot eyes approaches me as I leave my downtown Memphis office building. He says he needs money for the bus. I suspect he is instead trying to meet the price of a bottle of wine.

My defenses go up and I instinctively feel disdain for this fellow. It seems so obvious that he is wasting his life. How sad that he hasn't been able to pull himself together the way I did. I draw back as he offers to shake my hand.

What should I do next? The best thing is for me to try to be compassionate. First I will struggle to withhold my judgment. No one sets out to have a life like he has now. His name is Bill, by the way. Like you and me, he has an eternal soul.

I have no better idea about how Bill got here than he has about how I did. For all I know he is an army veteran, holder of a Distinguished Service Cross earned in Iraq, and suffering from hereditary mental illness exacerbated by PTSD. For all he knows, my expensive suit is a sign that I am a successful producer of pornography.

Let me struggle to remind myself that the fact that I am dressed better than Bill means my clothing is better than his. Not that I am better. The fact that I speak better than he does means I am more eloquent, not superior. The fact that I drink Sauvignon Blanc and Bill drinks Wild Irish Rose means I buy higher quality wine, not that I am higher quality. I am wealthier than Bill. That means only that I have more money.

First, then, let me withhold judgment of this man.

Second, let me treat him with respect. I won't give him money, but I will look him in the eye and greet him. I will address him as "Sir."

Respect has high value to Bill right now. Respect has high value to everyone, always.

Our compassion helps others. But why is compassion good for *me?* How will it make *me* more courageous?

Because perhaps if I learn to withhold judgment on others, I will learn to withhold judgment on myself. Perhaps if I treat others with respect, I will learn to treat myself that way. Perhaps the courage to love others will become the courage to love myself.

Despite your best intentions, you can't always be wise or helpful about what someone else needs. But you can always be compassionate: You can always be respectful of other people and their struggles. This will help you offer the same respect to yourself.

Let's not try to be heroes. Let's not try to be swimsuit models. Like Gene Kranz's engineers managing the *Apollo* 13 crisis, let's try to be better versions of what we already are. Let's do our best. That's good enough. That's plenty.

Many of our bad habits, our constantly repeating mistakes, are strategies to avoid short-term suffering. This is misguided. Trying to avoid suffering at all costs deprives you of creative suffering and the growth in personal power it produces. Also, life has a "pay me now or pay me later" quality. If you try to avoid suffering in the short term, you will suffer more down the road.

Where there is avoidance of suffering there is loss of courage, and where there is loss of courage there is no gumption. Where there is no gumption, there is no growth. Choose courage. Suffer better.

FUNDAMENTALS of
BETTER SUFFERING

1. You are going to suffer in this life. Choose suffering that builds courage.
2. Suffer not over things you can't control.
3. Flogging will not improve morale.
4. Beware of shortcuts. There are no helicopter rides on the mountain you are climbing.
5. Sometimes you have to turn and fight.
6. Holding a grudge is suffering needlessly by doing further damage to yourself.
7. Compassion for others will give you compassion for yourself.

GUMPTIONWORK

Today's Creative Suffering Menu

You can also do this online:
www.gumptionade.com/creative-suffering

Every day for a month, if you please: Choose one from Column A, one from Column B, and one from Column C. Please do not choose things that are in your comfort zone already (for example, "No smoking" does not represent suffering for me). You can add your own Creative Suffering options in the Reader's Choice boxes.

A PHYSICAL SUFFERING	B EMOTIONAL DISCOMFORT	C DEPRIVATION
Eat sashimi, chicken feet, or some other delicacy that makes you anxious.	Express your feelings to someone you admire.	No booze.
Take the stairs.	The next time you are angry take ten deep breaths and see how you feel.	No gossip.
Keep your thermostat three degrees off what you like.	Admit a wrong, and apologize for it.	No smoking.
Fast.	Sing to somebody.	Go to bed hungry.
Downward dog.	Ask someone way out of your league to lunch.	No music.

GUMPTIONWORK

A	B	C
PHYSICAL SUFFERING	**EMOTIONAL DISCOMFORT**	**DEPRIVATION**
Scrub the floor.	Find three reasons to like that person who annoys you.	No snacks.
Twenty push-ups.	Talk to people you don't know in the elevator.	No TV or video.
Take a cold shower.	Express sincere appreciation for criticism.	No meat.
Get up an hour early.	Converse with a very young child, listening closely.	No caffeine.
Reader's Choice	Reader's Choice	Reader's Choice
Reader's Choice	Reader's Choice	Reader's Choice
Reader's Choice	Reader's Choice	Reader's Choice
Reader's Choice	Reader's Choice	Reader's Choice

FUNDAMENTALS
of COURAGE

1. Know what Courage is for:

    a. Right after you get hit in the
        mouth (aka Day 4)
    b. Harmless things that scare you
        so bad you hurt yourself
    c. So *Regret* and *Shame* can't hide
        the lessons of failure
    d. When the status quo persecutes you
    e. So you have common sense and
        resourcefulness when it counts
    f. Bearing the discomfort that
        comes with real change.

2. Put excellence before success.
3. Translate uncertainty into risk.
4. Choose suffering that makes you more than
    you are now.
5. Don't stop for coffee when you are walking
    through Hell.

III
HOW TO BE
RESOURCEFUL

Chapter 10

LOOK FOR THE
FORCE OF THINGS

*There must be a drawing power
in matter...Therefore the apple
draws the earth, as well as
the earth draws the apple."*
ISAAC NEWTON

O
N A SUNNY SEVENTEENTH CENTURY
afternoon in Lincolnshire, England, Isaac Newton saw an apple fall from a tree and asked himself
why it didn't fall *up*. He was working out the force of things.

Being a colossal genius, Newton supplied his own answer:
"Assuredly, the reason is that the earth draws it." Newton then
discovered a set of facts — the force of gravity and the laws of
motion — that improved his understanding of how things work,
including the orbit of the moon around the earth.

Newton was resourceful. He looked for the force of things
behind an everyday occurrence. He discovered facts that
changed his understanding of the universe. If *you* look for the

force of things behind everyday occurrences, you'll discover facts that change your understanding of *your* universe. You will discover why you do things you wish you wouldn't.

Have you felt free all these years, free to make choices big and small, confident you were not influenced or coerced? You have in fact been subject to the force of things. Your judgment and decision making have been pushed and pulled by invisible forces, some benign and some not. The latter have sometimes prevented you from acting rationally, from being resourceful on your own behalf.

Seneca asked, "What is drunkenness other than insanity purposefully assumed?" Let us expand on this:

- Is it possible that habitual procrastination is mediocre performance purposefully assumed?
- What force could make someone accept the ill health and unattractiveness of obesity?
- Can tardiness ever be a way of expressing contempt?
- Is there something other than sexual desire that makes someone accept the risk of dishonor and disease that accompanies promiscuity?
- When could chronic disorganization be interpreted as confusion purposefully assumed?

There is an invisible force of things in your life. Look for it behind the choices you make.

I know something about you, my friend, whether you are a stranger, my reader, my neighbor, or my editor: Once upon a time, somewhere, someplace, you were a child.

> *There was a child went forth every day;*
> *And the first object he look'd upon...*
> *Became part of him for the day...or for many years...*
> *His own parents...*
> *They gave this child more of themselves than that;*
> *They gave him afterward every day—*
> *they became part of him.*
>
> Walt Whitman

The human psyche grows like a tree, adding new rings around previous growth. Every day you live becomes a part of who you are and how you think. No matter how tall and mighty you grow, however, The Child You Were remains at the core. Your childhood is a powerful force of things in your adult life.

During the time of the Trojan Wars, King Telephus of Mysia (now part of Turkey) was speared in the thigh by Achilles. Over time, the quarrel between the Mysians and the Greeks healed over. The king's wound did not. It caused him great pain.

Telephus questioned the Oracle at Delphi as to how he

might recover the use of his leg. The oracle answered "he that wounded shall heal." Scrapings from the point of Achilles's spear were applied to the wound, and it did heal.

Many adults carry an unhealed wound from childhood that weakens their ability to think and act resourcefully. They are aware of the discomfort, but unlike Telephus, they are not aware of the source.

> *From the child of five to myself is but a step. But from the new-born baby to the child of five is an appalling distance.*
>
> LEO TOLSTOY

In his 1954 book *Motivation and Personality*, psychologist Abraham Maslow explained the primary importance to each of us of meeting our basic requirements for survival: food, water, warmth, security, and affiliation.

At some early point in their lives, all children realize they cannot meet these needs without the help of adults. Combine this with the fact that young children cannot establish — let alone enforce — effective physical or emotional boundaries. You get resentment in the best of childhoods, confusion and terror in the worst.

In *Our Inner Conflicts*, psychiatrist Karen Horney called the latter situation the source of "The basic anxiety…a feeling the child has of being isolated and helpless in a potentially hostile world."

Deprivation, domination, abandonment, and domestic violence create chaos for some children. The unluckiest of them also lack alternative support networks among family or friends. Chaotic environments are stressful for an adult. They are harder still on children. Childhood — the place where Santa Claus and the Easter Bunny live and work — is a low-validity environment.

Low-validity environments give false positives, teach wicked lessons: You can't do things right. You deserve this punishment. It will teach you a lesson. This is how adults behave!

Children can be overexposed to stress at a time when they and their reasoning are small and weak. They will struggle to protect themselves.

Horney described that struggle: "Harassed by these disturbing conditions, the child gropes for ways to keep going, to cope with this menacing world. Despite his own weakness and fears, he unconsciously shapes his tactics to meet the particular forces operating in his environment. In doing so he develops not only ad hoc strategies, but *lasting character trends* which become part of his personality."

Children's brains are undeveloped. Their ad hoc strategies are not robust. My childhood strategy for dealing with my bedtime fear of monsters was to pull the covers over my head. St. Paul wrote to the people of Corinth, "When I was a child, I talked like a child, I thought like a child, I reasoned like a child." So did you.

Looking for the force that caused his irrational fear of public speaking, psychologist Allen Wheelis recalled a childhood marred by arbitrary cruelties packaged by his father as lessons.

To punish Allen for a poor grade at school, his father forced him to spend one summer cutting the lawn with a straight razor.

Little Allen learned a lesson from that, all right, but it was the wrong lesson: Because he could not measure up to his father's impossible standards, he was not good enough. After a great deal of hard work, grown-up Allen eventually discovered and wrote about the invisible emotional force transmitted from childhood: "What has made my father's voice so irresistible all these years, his judgment of me so implacably my destiny, has been the continuing silent and unnoticed reception of his message."

By finally "noticing" the message he was receiving unawares, Wheelis could then answer the question: What force prevents me from speaking in public? That brought options for doing better, for being more.

The Adverse Childhood Experiences (ACE) Study was conducted among 17,000 mostly middle-class Americans in the 1990s. It proved that children exposed to high levels of stress at home were much more likely than other children to have learning and behavioral problems in school, and chronic depression, alcoholism, drug abuse, smoking, and obesity as adults.

The key sources of childhood stress were household dysfunction, abuse, and neglect.

Recent advances in neurobiology have provided physical proof that severe stress changes the structure of a healthy childhood brain. The developing neural pathways and hormonal systems that make up a normal stress response system become hyperactive and stay that way. Adult symptoms parallel those of post-traumatic stress disorder in soldiers: anger, depression, hypervigilance, and avoidant behaviors. Resourceful behaviors like controlling impulses and forming healthy relationships are difficult.

Do you want to understand why someone repeatedly acts without common sense in some important aspect of their adult life? Why some people cannot control their behavior, their eating, their drinking, their spending, their acting out? Look to the past. Look for the outmoded survival strategies of confused children and their hairy ancestors. Look for behaviors that made sense once, but don't work now. Look for the visible footprints of invisible reference points.

The Child You Were is a force of things in your life.

Financial incentives are another powerful force of things. There are few better predictors of why an adult or an organization does what they do.

The American Coalition for Clean Coal Electricity cannot understand the benefits of a U.S. energy policy that puts limits on carbon emissions. Why ? Because, as Upton Sinclair wrote, "It is difficult to get a man to understand something, when his salary depends upon his not understanding it."

The American Coalition for Clean Coal Electricity may be right, they may be wrong, but if you follow the money you will understand the incentive for them to want what they want:

- Reason #1: The Coalition is funded by coal producers and the railroads that ship coal.
- Reason #2: Burning coal creates significantly more carbon emissions than burning natural gas, its primary competitor for the business of electricity-generating power plants.

You could discuss the unanswered questions about clean coal and the threat of climate change with the president of the American Coalition for Clean Coal Electricity. No matter how many facts you have, though, he will not understand why natural gas is superior to coal for electricity generation. His salary depends upon his not understanding it. If I had his job and paycheck, I wouldn't either.

What incentive did the Tobacco Institute have for arguing so strenuously for so many years against the growing body of scientific proof about the dangers of smoking? Start here: Their money came from tobacco companies.

A recent study published in the *British Journal of Medicine* questions the efficacy of annual mammograms in reducing deaths from breast cancer. The study has been harshly criticized by the American College of Radiology and the Society of Breast Imaging.

These two fine organizations may be right. Listen to their arguments before you decide about annual mammograms. But also follow the money. The American College of Radiology and the Society of Breast Imaging are both organized and funded by people who make their living from mammography. It is impossible for them to view the recent study in an impartial light.

On any issue of importance, look for the incentives behind someone's point of view. Look for your own. It won't always be money, of course. Other powerful incentives include security, comfort, and sex.

Gravity is an underlying force of things in the universe. Incentives are an underlying force of things in human affairs. Don't ask a barber whether you need a haircut.

You have a unique set of reasons why you want what you want. Unlike those of the American Coalition for Clean Coal Electricity, many of your incentives are difficult for you to see.

Isaac Newton saw the invisible force of gravity and translated it into a law of the universe that changed science. Alan Wheelis saw the invisible force of a wicked lesson he learned in childhood, bringing it into consciousness in a way that changed his life.

How can you make discoveries about the invisible forces operating in your own life? By looking for causes, exploring the people and events, past and present, that may be influencing you; by listening for the messages you receive unawares about who you are, what you can and can't do, should and shouldn't be. Some of these are unnoticed messages from The Child You Were and from Your Hairy Ancestor. Some are loud and clear from those in the present who either actively wish ill for you or simply don't know how hurtful their remarks are. Some are subliminal messages delivered by marketing companies to convince you to buy things that you don't need.

Start by observing everyday facts about yourself and asking simple questions about what force makes you do what you do. Perhaps one of these might resemble a question below:

- The fact is that I want to be more disciplined about my work, but I don't follow through. What force is resisting that?
- The fact is I weigh seventy pounds more than I want to. Why? What is causing this?
- The fact is that I want to start my own business, but I always delay. What force is pushing against my desire?
- The fact is that I need to save money for my retirement, but I never do. What's going on?
- The fact is I drank 180 beers last month when I intended to drink none. Why? What force is acting on me?
- The fact is I am lonely, but I don't try to make friends. What's happening here?
- The fact is that I scream at my children, even though it makes me feel bad. Why?
- The fact is I sleep with people I don't love, and then regret it. What force is at work?
- (Reader's Choice) The fact is I _____ _____.

    What force is at work here?

What is the force pushing back against your best intentions? What weighs you down so, on Day Four? What are the things that scare you so bad you hurt yourself? Try to avoid easy answers, including but not limited to: "It's not my fault," or "It's all my fault." Don't guess. Know.

If something causes one effect it may cause other, bigger effects. The force that makes an apple fall also makes the moon orbit the earth. The force that inflames my anger at the person ahead of me in the "10 Items or Less" line — the scoundrel has thirteen — is also limiting my income by making me difficult to work with.

Knowledge is power. Once we know that malaria is spread by mosquitoes, we know how to avoid it. If we know why a plane crashed, we can become safer in the air. If I know why I am so easy to anger, I might see how to overcome my bad temper. Just seeing clearly that I *am* bad-tempered makes me better than I was.

The force of things: Invisible gravity encourages the attraction of objects; invisible bacteria in drinking water encourages illness; invisible damage from emotions experienced in childhood encourages wasteful adult behaviors.

Understanding the force of things in your life will make you more resourceful. Being resourceful is a key to gumption, to do what needs to be done.

FUNDAMENTALS of
the FORCE of THINGS

1. You are subject to the force of things.
2. Gravity is an invisible force that influences the behavior of objects large and small.
3. The Child You Were is an invisible force that influences your adult behavior.
4. Your Hairy Ancestor is an invisible force that influences your adult behavior.
5. Financial incentives are an invisible force that influence everyone's adult behavior.

GUMPTIONWORK

Childhood Stress Calibration Tool

You can do this better online:
www.gumptionade.com/childhood-stress

Do you think you may have had a too stressful childhood? If you answer yes to any of the questions below, you may have. (If you were not raised by your parents, simply use "parents" to mean "the people who raised me.")

For a formal review of the ACE study and questionnaire, on which I based this work sheet, see the ACE Study pages at the Centers for Disease Control and Prevention websites (cdc.gov/ace/index.htm) and a condensed questionnaire and discussion at http://acestoohigh.com/got-your-ace-score/.

	YES	NO
One or both of my parents was an alcoholic or a drug addict when I was a child.	☐	☐
An outside observer might say that I was frequently hit by a parent when I was a child.	☐	☐
An outside observer might say I was sexually abused when I was a child.	☐	☐
An outside observer might say that I was emotionally abused when I was a child.	☐	☐
One or both of my parents was chronically ill or died when I was a child.	☐	☐
One or both of my parents was wildly unpredictable when I was a child, and not always in a good way.	☐	☐
I was chronically ill when I was a child.	☐	☐

GUMPTIONWORK

	YES	NO
My parents divorced when I was less than seven years old.	☐	☐
My family or I moved more than five times before I was seven.	☐	☐
I witnessed physical violence in my home when I was a child.	☐	☐

The question may not be, "What's wrong with you?" It may be: "What did you go through?"

_____

_____

_____

_____

_____

_____

_____

_____

_____

_____

_____

_____

Chapter 11

PULL UP THE ANCHOR BEFORE YOU ADD SAIL

"Man muss immer umkehren"

(Invert, always invert)

<small>MATHEMATICIAN CARL JACOBI
(EXPRESSING THE IDEA THAT MANY HARD PROBLEMS
CAN BE SOLVED BY TURNING THEM UPSIDE DOWN)</small>

"I F MY JOB WAS TO PICK A GROUP OF TEN stocks in the Dow Jones Industrial Average that would outperform the average itself," Warren Buffett once said, "I would try to pick the ten or fifteen worst performers and take them out of the sample and work with the residual." He inverts to solve a hard problem. Buffett starts towards success by first noticing and removing failure.

You are the captain of your ship. For heaven's sake, pull up your anchor before you add more sail.

You want to make more money? Look first at how to spend *less*. Making more money depends a great deal on factors outside of your control. Spending less does not. Start there.

You want to lose weight? Look first at how you gain weight. Do you eat too much when you are upset? Do you drink soda? Do you require that dieting be painless? Start your weight-losing plan by identifying and removing your worst weight-gaining behaviors.

You want your best customers to spend more? Look first at how to prevent them from spending *less*. Find out what they *don't* like about doing business with you and remove that. *Then* add things they might buy.

How can you find someone to love you? Start by removing the things that make you hard to love.

Invert your normal behavior. Instead of looking for what *might* work, look for what *hasn't*. Look for the predictable causes of failure. Start with a To-Don't list. Weigh anchor before you add sail.

Much is said about how to be happy. Practice your faith. Spend time with people who care about you. Cultivate a hobby. Help somebody. Laugh more.

Good ideas, all. But the fastest way to be happy is to remove something from your life that makes you unhappy.

Competitive cyclists know that the fastest way to increase speed is to lighten their bicycle or lighten themselves. First lose weight, *then* work on adding muscle power.

It is more resourceful to identify and remove recurring failure in your own behavior than try to copy the success of others. Here are some candidates for removal:

Nine Reliable Ways to Be Miserable

1. Bring ill health upon yourself
2. Commute a long way to work by automobile
3. Worry about things you can't control
4. Never be wrong
5. Don't forgive yourself or anybody else
6. Live for praise or gratitude
7. Don't get really good at some little thing
8. Spread yourself a mile wide and an inch deep
9. Covet what you don't need

Life will deliver you a portion of misery. Minimizing self-inflicted misery is a good way to be happier.

> "I hate to lose worse than anyone, but if you never lose, you won't know how to act."
>
> BEAR BRYANT

What would you do if I strapped you inside an aluminum tube and hurled you through the sky at five hundred miles an hour? That is to say, what would you do if I put you on a commercial airline flight?

In general terms, you would be aware of the complexity of the system that carries you and all that cargo so high, far, and fast. You would also be aware of the effect of gravity if things go wrong. So how is it that you can nap, catch up on work, read a magazine? Why aren't you a nervous wreck?

Because your chances of dying while traveling by domestic commercial flight are one in seven million. You are much more likely to be hit by lightning.

Frosted Pop-Tarts notwithstanding, the most successful industrial effort in America over the last hundred years has been the work of flying humans from point A to point B without dashing them into the ground.

This achievement comes from inverting, turning normal organizational behavior — trumpeting success and ignoring failure — on its head. The airplane manufacturers, the airlines, the National Transportation Safety Board, and the Federal Aviation Administration rigorously analyze failure. Then they publish what they learn.

Commercial airplanes have two black boxes operating at all times, a voice and a data recorder. They capture the who, what, when, and how of failure.

Experts descend upon a crash site by the hundreds to retrieve the black boxes, from mountain peak or ocean floor if necessary, and piece together the remnants of the plane.

They spend no time celebrating the success of the 99.99 percent of the flights that did not crash that day. The experts invert normal behavior. They look for the facts produced by failure — the facts about why this flying system broke down.

The FAA and the NTSB then require all involved to follow Alcoholics Anonymous step number five: "Admit to God, to ourselves, and to another human being the exact nature of our wrongs."

The crash of American Airlines Flight 191 in May of 1979 was the worst air disaster in U.S. history. Here is a summary of the facts uncovered *and published* by the National Transportation Safety Board:

> The probable cause of this accident was…maintenance-induced damage leading to the separation of the No. 1 engine and pylon assembly at a critical point during takeoff…Contributing to the cause of the accident were the vulnerability of the design of the pylon attach points to maintenance damage…Federal Aviation Administration surveillance and reporting systems which failed…practices and communications among the operators, the manufacturer, and the FAA which failed.

The number one engine fell off the plane during takeoff. The cause was a combination of design mistakes, damage in maintenance, and poor communications. Everyone was told. It never happened again.

Don't guess about your failures. Know.

There were less than two hundred U.S. commercial airline fatalities in the *ten years* ending with 2012. A commercial airline flight is safer than it really ought to be.

You know what isn't? U.S. hospital care. A recent study in the *Journal of Patient Safety* estimated there are over 200,000 preventable deaths of hospital patients *every year*.

Would you be surprised to learn that hospitals, physicians, medical manufacturers, and government agencies do not jointly investigate these failures and publish what they learn? That they bury their mistakes?

Would you be surprised to learn that physicians are less concerned than airline pilots about fatal accidents?

Would you be surprised to learn that physicians often base their diagnostic and treatment decisions on their own experience and preference, rather than on available statistics? That financial incentives play a role?

There is increasing pressure on U.S. hospitals and physicians to practice evidence-based medicine. There is no pressure for evidence-based commercial aviation. We already have it.

If you want to fly better, invert normal human behavior. Record failure with black box rigor. Study it, and shout what you learn from the mountaintops.

If you want to *be* better, invert *your* normal behavior. Analyze your own failures. Do what you can to live an evidence-based life. Simple. Not easy.

Nobel Prize-winning physicist Niels Bohr called an expert someone "who has made all the mistakes which can be made, in a very narrow field." Failure is not just the best teacher. Failure is the only teacher. If you have not failed at something, you don't know much about it.

Success depends on a long chain of interrelated circumstances and often includes a significant amount of luck. Like Nassim Taleb's Wall Street Magoos, you can be right for the wrong reasons. Success looks inevitable after the fact.

That illusion also makes it seem possible to know the real cause of success: the brilliant leader, the great talent, the huge budget. Important factors in achieving success, all of them, but not necessarily decisive. Few things are more random than weather, for example, and weather can be crucial.

The largest amphibious assault in history began in the pre-dawn hours of June 6, 1944. The Allied invasion of Normandy called for training, equipping, and transporting soldiers, sailors, and airmen on a scale never before attempted. They fought with initiative and courage. It is one of the great military successes of all time.

It almost didn't come off. On June 4, 1944, the worst storm in the English Channel in decades made it impossible to launch the invasion force on either June 5 or the June 6 backup day. The operation would have to be delayed until the time of the next full moon and favorable tides.

The 184,000 Allied troops and their 5,000 ships were at embarkation points or already in the Channel. The second wave of men and material was filling the just-vacated beds and berths. A month's delay meant the German army in France would see all this activity.

The disastrous weather threatened the Normandy invasion and the career of Dwight Eisenhower, the Commander of the Allied Expeditionary Force.

Eisenhower scrubbed June 5. On that day a high-pressure ridge unexpectedly appeared from the west that promised to temporarily push out the storm conditions. Based on the forecast for barely favorable weather on the sixth, Eisenhower gave the orders to proceed.

He was brave and he was lucky. Not only did the day clear up enough to make the invasion possible, but the terrible weather that immediately preceded it caused some of the German troops to stand down. Many officers left for the weekend, including their commander, Erwin Rommel. By midnight on June 6, the Allies had established themselves along a fifty-mile front on the coast of Normandy.

Germany surrendered ten months later. Eisenhower went on to become the thirty-fourth president of the United States. Weather.

A successful person, team, company, or nation may appear to have been destined for that outcome, but success is inscrutable. The illusion of inevitability disguises the crucial role of chance in the unfolding of events.

The great paradox of life is that failure is the source of progress. Indeed, the idea that wisdom, love, and power will spring up in unlikely places is fundamental to the stories of all civilizations. Nature grows roses in dirt and dung.

Jesus Christ had failure written all over him. He came from Nazareth — the Camden, New Jersey, of its day. He was born in a cave. He owned no land, the mark of powerlessness in that era. He was unemployed. Why would the Jewish establishment think Jesus was the messiah whose arrival the prophets had foretold?

He had a few troublesome and disloyal followers, not powerful legions. He died a criminal's death, abandoned, not the attended passing of a great man. Yet what was Caesar compared to Christ?

Progress usually comes from the wrong side of the tracks, from the border lands. Like the personal computer (a garage). Like penicillin (a brewery). Like sabermetrics (baseball fans). Like the Beatles (Liverpool). Like Christianity.

What good can come from Nazareth? What good can come from *your* failures? Only what you need to become better: facts and options.

American scholar Joseph Campbell found common ground in the mythology of cultures worldwide. A universal metaphor is life represented as a physical journey from home to a new place. We moderns have inherited the journeys of Gilgamesh, Odysseus, Jonah, Percival, Red Riding Hood, Dante, Huck Finn, and Frodo Baggins.

A common feature is the presence of fearsome border guardians, ready to turn back the unprepared, frightened, or unlucky traveler.

To begin their voyage for the Golden Fleece, the Argonauts had to first pass through the Symplegades, a pair of massive rocks that clashed together randomly, threatening to crush them before they could get to open water.

Dragons guard the doors of temples, standing between us and the treasure inside.

Campbell wrote about one border guardian, the classical Greek god Pan. Pan patrolled the area beyond the boundary of civilization and might cast a spell of fatal dread — panic — onto humans who accidentally crossed that threshold. *But* Pan yielded good health and wisdom to travelers who approached him in an intentional and respectful manner. Be mindful of this on Day Four.

You know there are obstacles on your path. Your recurring failures, your bad habits — these are the demons guarding your boundaries, preventing you from moving forward. They come in different sizes, depending on the power of the knowledge they guard: small and nettlesome ("Why do I always lose my keys?"); large and deadly ("Why can't I stop drinking?").

Your fears — of failure, rejection, shame — are great. Your fears stand between you and the person you want to be. They also clarify things. As soon as you see these demons, you know where you need to go — beyond them. Simple. Not easy.

Sometimes your border guardian looks ridiculous. Had Shakespeare's King Lear listened to his fool, he would never have divided his kingdom among his fawning daughters. He would never have banished Cordelia, the daughter who spoke honestly and loved him truly.

KING LEAR: When were you wont to be so full of songs, sirrah?
FOOL: I have used it, nuncle, ever since thou madest thy
daughters thy mothers: For when thou gavest them
the rod and put'st down thine own breeches,
[Singing] Then they for sudden joy did weep, and I for sorrow sung.

Invert: The Fool is wise and the king is foolish. The Fool—your foolish self, your failure—will show you what you need to know, if you can bear to pay attention. You are more likely to look away. It is humiliating to admit you were wrong, you were weak. It is also resourceful, for that is where your power lies.

Your company's famous bleu cheese has turned noir by the time it arrives at Costco. Investigation reveals inaccurate shipping labels. Misaddressed shipments, it turns out, shine a light on inadequate software training in the warehouse. Where else will this training issue cause failure? More light, better vision, more facts.

Your beloved apple tree—the one your grandfather planted, the one you climbed many a happy day as a child—falls over in a violent windstorm. Weep, of course. Curse if you must. But pick the apples.

You are shipwrecked on a deserted Caribbean island. Swim out to the wreck, Robinson Crusoe, and salvage the tools and weapons you need to survive, before your broken ship sinks out of sight.

Your advertising agency goes belly up. Overrule your wounded ego and run a secondhand office equipment sale to get the cash you need to survive the next few months.

Follow Jacobi's advice and invert to solve a hard problem: Mine your failures for gold. Turn your demons and fools into guides for your journey to a new and better place.

How to be more resourceful, how to have more gumption, is a hard problem. Invert. Weigh anchor before adding sail. Before you spend time and money trying to obtain tools and talents that will make you more successful, examine what you do that makes you *less.*

Please don't ignore failure because it's embarrassing. Your own mistakes are the evidence you need to live an evidence-based life. Pay black box attention. Demand recompense. Accept nothing less than facts and options.

The world really needs to know the seven habits of highly *ineffective* people, so we can start by removing them.

FUNDAMENTALS
of INVERTING

1. Pull up anchor before adding sail.
2. Success is a poor teacher.
3. Breakthroughs come from the wrong side of the tracks.
4. Hindsight is blind to the role of randomness.
5. Listen to your Fool.
6. Pick the apples before you chop up the fallen tree.

GUMPTIONWORK

Failure
Calibration
Tool

You can do this better online:
www.gumptionade.com/failure-calibration

How we create more success in our lives is a hard problem.
Let us invert the problem and make it easier: How can we
create less failure? The best way to start is to identify and
remove it from our lives.

Your bad habits are recurring failures that lower your
gumption. Some bad habits — say, a weakness for clut-
ter — are regrettable but don't do heavy damage. Others are
downright toxic to gumption and must be mapped.

Please write your worst habit here:

_____

_____

Please answer the following yes or no questions:

1. Do you try to hide this bad habit?
   ☐ Yes ☐ No
2. Do you wonder if you have a problem?
   ☐ Yes ☐ No
3. Do you feel uneasy when resisting this habit?
   ☐ Yes ☐ No
4. Is this bad habit a means of feeling better when
   having a bad day?
   ☐ Yes ☐ No

GUMPTIONWORK

5. Does your habit take too much of your time, or your money, or your thoughts?
☐ Yes ☐ No
6. Do you feel guilty after you engage in this habit but do it again soon?
☐ Yes ☐ No
7. Do you make promises to yourself about this habit and then break them?
☐ Yes ☐ No
8. Do you continue your habit, even though it causes health problems?
☐ Yes ☐ No

Bonus questions for readers whose bad habit is drinking:
9. Have you said the words "road beer" in the last month?
☐ Yes ☐ No
10. Have you ever had a blackout caused by drinking?
☐ Yes ☐ No
11. Have you lost your keys/wallet/phone in the past twenty-four months?
☐ Yes ☐ No
12. Have you switched to vodka?
☐ Yes ☐ No

Every yes answer is worth one point. If you scored two points or higher, you may have a dangerous habit. Welcome to the club. You will likely need WhoHowness to deal with it. Consider talking to a mental health professional. If you are a drinker, consider AA.

For the rest of you, what golden apples are your demons guarding?

Chapter 12

FRAME YOUR
DECISIONS

In the land of the blind, the
one-eyed man is king.

Desiderius Erasmus

O N October 30, 1935, Boeing's new
four-engine bomber began its demonstration flight
at Wilbur Wright Field. The A299 was favored
to become the Army Air Force's next generation long range
bomber. The plane rolled powerfully down the runway, took
off, and climbed rapidly. Then it stalled, fell to the earth, and
exploded.

The cause was an error by the pilot, the chief of flight testing. While seeing to the large number of takeoff procedures
required by this advanced airplane, neither he nor his copilot
remembered to unlock the rudder controls. Human judgment
is unreliable. It can fail at crucial times.

The A299 outstripped the ability of pilots to execute
required procedures in proper order. After the crash, it was

considered too complicated to fly safely. The contract went to the Douglas DB-1, which later proved unsatisfactory for combat operations.

Boeing's airplane was so much better, however, that a loophole in contracting specifications was used to equip one squadron. The Air Force named it the B-17. A reporter called it the Flying Fortress.

B-17s eventually flew thousands of precision-bombing attacks on German military-industrial capacity during World War II. The plane achieved iconic status for allowing American crews to complete missions despite sustaining heavy damage from enemy antiaircraft and fighters.

How did the risky A299 become the dependable B-17? Because the airplane was *not* too complicated to fly safely. It was too complicated to fly safely without help. There were too many things to remember.

B-17 pilots needed visible reference points. They needed a written checklist so they could *see* all the procedures for flying the plane. By March of 1944, the checklist looked like the one opposite this page.

Checklists are now part of standard operating procedure for flying any aircraft.

You have a mission every day: to do what needs to be done. You have work and family obligations. You have an obligation to yourself, to become more than you are now. There are distractions. Like B-17 pilots, your memory is unreliable. In addition, you lack an instrument panel and a copilot. Make a checklist.

APPROVED B-17F and G CHECKLIST

REVISED 3-1-44

PILOT'S DUTIES IN RED
COPILOT'S DUTIES IN BLACK

BEFORE STARTING
1. Pilot's Preflight—COMPLETE
2. Form 1A—CHECKED
3. Controls and Seats—CHECKED
4. Fuel Transfer Valves & Switch—OFF
5. Intercoolers—Cold
6. Gyros—UNCAGED
7. Fuel Shut-off Switches—OPEN
8. Gear Switch—NEUTRAL
9. Cowl Flaps—Open Right—
   OPEN LEFT—Locked
10. Turbos—OFF
11. Idle cut-off—CHECKED
12. Throttles—CLOSED
13. High RPM—CHECKED
14. Autopilot—OFF
15. De-icers and Anti-icers, Wing and
    Prop—OFF
16. Cabin Heat—OFF
17. Generators—OFF

STARTING ENGINES
1. Fire Guard and Call Clear—LEFT Right
2. Master Switch—ON
3. Battery switches and inverters—ON &
   CHECKED
4. Parking Brakes—Hydraulic Check—On-
   CHECKED
5. Booster Pumps—Pressure—ON &
   CHECKED
6. Carburetor Filters—Open
7. Fuel Quantity—Gallons per tank
8. Start Engines: both magnetos on
   after one revolution
9. Flight Indicator & Vacuum Pressures
   CHECKED
10. Radio—On
11. Check Instruments CHECKED
12. Crew Report
13. Radio Call & Altimeter—SET

ENGINE RUN-UP
1. Brakes—Locked
2. Trim Tabs—SET
3. Exercise Turbos and Props
4. Check Generators—CHECKED & OFF
5. Run up Engines

BEFORE TAKEOFF
1. Tailwheel—Locked
2. Gyro—Set
3. Generators—ON

AFTER TAKEOFF
1. Wheel—PILOT'S SIGNAL
2. Power Reduction
3. Cowl Flaps
4. Wheel Check—OK right—OK LEFT

BEFORE LANDING
1. Radio Call, Altimeter—SET
2. Crew Positions—OK
3. Autopilot—OFF
4. Booster Pumps—On
5. Mixture Controls—AUTO-RICH
6. Intercooler—Set
7. Carburetor Filters—Open
8. Wing De-icers Off
9. Landing Gear
   a. Visual—Down Right—DOWN LEFT
      Tailwheel Down, Antenna in, Ball
      Turret Checked
   b. Light—OK
   c. Switch Off—Neutral
10. Hydraulic Pressure—OK Valve closed
11. RPM 2100—Set
12. Turbos—Set
13. Flaps ⅓—⅓ Down

FINAL APPROACH
14. Flaps—PILOT'S SIGNAL
15. RPM 2200—PILOT'S SIGNAL

Page one of the B-17 checklist that hung by a lanyard on the back of the pilot's seat in 1944.

Let's say that your commitment to personal growth requires eating sensibly and getting regular exercise. The checklist for your daily mission might look like this:

My Daily Mission Checklist

GROUP 1

☐ weigh myself and write down the number

☐ eat breakfast

☐ eat four servings of vegetables

☐ water, not soda

☐ wait twenty minutes before having seconds

☐ take a thirty-minute walk

☐ apple for dessert

GROUP 2

☐ make daily plan before starting work

☐ start with the #1 priority

☐ check in with boss

☐ review and respond to all messages

GROUP 3

☐ call spouse during the day to see how things are going for them

☐ review children's schoolwork before turning on the TV

☐ do one thing on the "little stuff" list

☐ read for pleasure

Pilots also have special checklists for emergencies — visible reference points for scary situations like a sudden loss of power or smoke in the cockpit.

We could all use better reference points during scary situations like bitter quarrels, family holidays, or a sudden, overwhelming need to do wrong things.

Economist and philosopher Vilfredo Pareto noted some facts about early-twentieth-century Italian agriculture. Looking at his nation, he noted that 20 percent of the population owned 80 percent of the land. Looking at his garden, he noted that 20 percent of the pea pods produced 80 percent of the peas. Pareto asked himself why this distribution applied to both the big and the small, the social and the vegetable. He looked for the force of it.

The principle that resulted, the Law of the Vital Few, has implications for your ability to do what needs to be done. You may have heard it called the 80/20 rule.

Twenty percent of anything will produce 80 percent of the results. Twenty percent of the beer drinkers will drink 80 percent of the beer. Twenty percent of the stocks in the S&P 500 will produce 80 percent of the returns. Twenty percent of software bugs produce 80 percent of the complaints.

Twenty percent of the things *you* do will generate 80 percent of your results. Whether your goal is a healthy weight, advancement at work, or finding a suitable mate, you can't do everything you'd like to do. You can't do everything people tell you to do. You have too much to look after every day. Look for the vital few things you *must* do to reach your goal.

The 80/20 Rule in Action

Who	The Vital Few Things	Not Vital
Gene Kranz	• Trajectory • Air speed • Battery charge • Oxygen levels	• Our science experiments • Whose fault is this? • Supply of Tang™
Billy Beane	• On-base percentage • Salary requirement	• Batting Average • Foot Speed • Good Looks
Ann Richards	• Number of alcoholic beverages consumed today	• What other people think of me • How funny I am • Happy Hour start time
John Snow	• Cholera deaths by street address • Source of drinking water by street address	• London air pollution • Color of the Thames • Number of cholera survivors

What are your vital few facts?

Simple formulas are more accurate than expert opinion, particularly in low-validity environments.

- A simple formula (high school grades and one aptitude test) was more accurate in predicting the grades of college freshman than were experienced counselors who had that information and much more.

- A simple formula using three facts about local weather is more accurate than wine experts in predicting the value of Bordeaux vintages.
- Simple formulas are more accurate than expert opinion for many other decisions, including the diagnosis of cardiac disease, evaluating credit risk, assessing foster parents, and predicting recidivism among juvenile offenders.

Simple formulas are more accurate because they use only the vital few facts. They do not depend on personal judgment, influenced as it is by emotions and the opinions of others. Guessing, even by experts, is not resourceful. Simple formulas reduce guessing. Don't guess. Know.

What simple formulas can you apply to your life? Here are a few:

Simple Formulas for Complex Problems

- Formula for losing weight: Calories consumed per week are less than calories needed to maintain current weight.
- Formula for increasing your vocabulary: Hours per day reading are greater than hours watching TV or video.
- Formula for getting rich over the long haul: Annual spending as a percentage of your annual income is less than ninety-one.

- Formula for lowering the risk of heart disease: Number of minutes per week exercising is at least one hundred eighty.
- Formula for avoiding insanity purposefully assumed: Beer consumed per hour is no more than twelve ounces.
- Formula for appearing wise: Ratio of time spent listening to time spent talking is 3:1.
- Formula for preventing divorce: Frequency of lovemaking is greater than frequency of fighting.

Why is it more difficult to make a forty-two-yard field goal in the last seconds of the Super Bowl than to make one on the practice field in August? The distance is the same. The football is the same. Yet the practice kick is trivial, while the Super Bowl–winning kick is a lasting triumph of skill and courage.

The reason is context. That is the only thing that has changed, and it has changed dramatically. The hopes and dreams of coaches and teammates, the $92,000 per player winners' bonus, a stadium full of screaming spectators, and a national television audience of 114 million people have ratcheted the consequences of success or failure up to the sky.

Context: a one-word description of the set of your reference points, everything that affects how you feel, how you think, and how you act: the roar of the crowd; your father's often-repeated opinions about you; the smell of cinnamon rolls baking; a gun pointed at your face; your parents' divorce; a hot bath; a cold beer; 3 a.m. anxiety; a tongue in your ear; transcendent music; the cry of your newborn child; forty-four reporters camped out in front of your office; the president calling on line one.

Some reference points are fleeting, some are engraved in stone. Some are easy to see and some are invisible. The collective human evolutionary experience (snake bad) and our own childhood experience (chicken soup good) also create visible and invisible reference points we carry in our heads.

One part of my childhood experience created a context that makes me oversensitive to criticism, irrationally afraid of being judged and found wanting. This has caused me problems.

One night long ago I learned I had been ridiculed by a fellow Kenyon student I barely knew and cared nothing about. I spent two fruitless hours walking around campus looking for him. I proved him right. My childish reference point led me astray.

On important matters, it is resourceful to take the time to identify misleading context and exclude it from your decision frame:

- "I won't retire for twenty years. I can buy the car I want now and be just as good as my brother-in-law." Can this decision frame be broadened to include better facts about the future?
- "I know I drink too much, but if I follow the Alcoholics Anonymous program I won't be able to make a champagne toast at my daughter's

wedding." Can this decision frame be narrowed
to focus on the here and now?

- "I know that I have always failed to lose weight
  and keep it off, but with Raspberry Ketones,
  this time is going to be different." Can this
  decision frame be broadened to include better
  facts from the past?
- "I don't understand what the lecturer means by
  Bayesian probability. It feels important, but if
  I ask another question everyone will think I'm
  stupid." Can this decision frame be narrowed
  to exclude what other people may think?

Focusing on the vital few facts builds a more effective decision frame:

- *Fact*: "This retirement calculator indicates I
  need to double my savings rate to be financially
  independent after age seventy-six. I'll feel
  awful if I have to take money from my children.
  Perhaps I can drive the old car another year or
  two." These vital facts create the option of a
  financially independent future.
- *Fact*: "My daughter is nine years old. What if
  I don't drink today and wait until her wedding
  day to decide about that champagne toast?"
  Facts create the option to stay sober today and —
  maybe — drink champagne in sixteen years.
- *Fact*: "I fail over and over with these magic

diets. Why would this be different? I really
should try something else. Maybe I'll go
to Weight Watchers. I've heard they have a
sensible program, and my best friend lost
twenty-two pounds several years ago and has
kept it off." These facts offer up the possibility
of sustainable weight loss.

- *Fact:* "The other students in the class won't be
taking the final exam for me. I need to pass
this course to get into grad school. I will ask my
question." These vital few facts bring the option
of getting a better grade.

"*You need this brain surgery* to continue to see. There is a
4 percent chance that the procedure will cause you to bleed
profusely out of your ears and die on the operating table."

"You need this brain surgery to avoid going blind. This surgery has a 96 percent survival rate."

Your decision frame is influenced by two kinds of context:

1. *how* the choice is presented, as above, and
2. your *personal* reference points (failing vision, for
   example, fear, or a distrust of authority figures).

On important choices, pay attention to both.

Male rats that have mated and show no further interest in sex get busy if a new female is introduced into their environment. A change of context releases latent desire. This is why divorce lawyers drive BMWs.

My friend experiences cold and wet weather when he runs during the winter. It does not diminish his happiness. Indeed, challenging conditions increase his sense of accomplishment. My friend does not relish cold and wet weather on his way to the dentist. There is no difference in the weather. The difference is reference points. The reference point of running produces latent courage that overcomes the effect of bad weather on his mood. The dentist? Not so much.

If the personal meaning of your activity is high, latent courage will help you bear discomfort. By the way, what could be more meaningful than the work you do to become more than you are now? And what could be more uncomfortable?

Psychotherapy, so helpful for so many in overcoming crippling habits, is above all the evaluation of the context provided by your personal reference points. You and your therapist undertake a sometimes boring and often painful archeological dig through your experiences, thoughts, and feelings.

You slowly learn to exclude misleading reference points from your decision frame. You become better at focusing on the vital few facts, the 20 percent that provide 80 percent of your results. You see the force of things.

Let's stop here and take a breath. Let's admit that life is too short to parse *every* decision. Save time and brain power for the important ones — have default decisions for simple, recurring situations. Here are some of mine:

Nine Default Decisions for Bob O'Connor

1. Never buy extended warranties.
2. Always address men I don't know as "Sir."
3. Never buy a stock based on a tip in the media.
4. Always weigh myself first thing in the morning.
5. Never eat white chocolate (all the calories and none of the chocolate).
6. Always have a book to read.
7. Never argue with clients.
8. Always overtip hotel maids.
9. Never buy hair care products I can't use in the shower.

It is resourceful to conserve brain power for the important choices, the choices about how to be more than you are now. That's not hair care.

Don't be a hero. An obese person who resolves to eat perfectly for the rest of her life is asking too much. She will not survive the battle. The man who can't be wrong paints a target on his chest. He will be picked off. Keep your pretty head low.

Gene Kranz never asked his engineers to be heroes. He asked them to be the best of who they already were, to work hard and bring him facts and options.

You can't boil the ocean. The context created by "the rest of my life" is ineffective. Doing better today, however, can be accomplished. The context of today is effective.

The battle to overcome bad habits — to be more — is most of all a battle for context, the daily discipline of remembering and acting on effective reference points. Be resourceful. Put the vital few facts within your decision frame. Make a checklist.

Our field goal kicker focuses on facts and brackets out the intimidating context: "Wind is blowing a bit from right to left… back two steps, over one…aim at right upright to allow for a moderate drift." He controls his reference points as best he can, kicks the football, and then joins the rest of us to watch what happens next.

FUNDAMENTALS *of* DECISION FRAMING

1. Use a checklist to remember what needs to be done.
2. Look for the vital few facts.
3. Simple formulas are resourceful for making complex decisions.
4. Be aware of context when you make an important choice.
5. A change in context can summon latent power.
6. Develop defaults for small decisions that recur frequently.

GUMPTIONWORK

Checklist Template

You can do this better online:
www.gumptionade.com/checklist-template

Group 1

My Self-Improvement Disciplines *(every day)*

☐ _____

☐ _____

☐ _____

☐ _____

Group 2

My Work-Life Disciplines *(every weekday)*

☐ _____

☐ _____

☐ _____

☐ _____

Group 3

My Personal-Life Disciplines
(weekdays or every day, as applicable)

☐ _____

☐ _____

☐ _____

☐ _____

My Vital
Few Facts

You can also do this online:
www.gumptionade.com/my-vital-few-facts

Please write down your Top 5 bad habits

Behavior #1 _____

Behavior #2 _____

Behavior #3 _____

Behavior #4 _____

Behavior #5 _____

Now pick the one that causes you 80 percent of the problems
you have reaching your goals. Write down this bad habit
again here:

_____

You know what to do next. Look for the force of it. Write
down your ideas here, if you please: _____

_____

_____

_____

_____

_____

HOW TO BE RESOURCEFUL

FUNDAMENTALS *of* RESOURCEFULNESS

1. Look for the force of things.
2. Financial incentives are a force of things.
3. Your childhood is a force of things in your adult life.
4. Pull up the anchor before you add sail.
5. Study failure.
6. Create a decision frame around the things you can control.
7. Make a checklist.
8. Focus on the vital few facts (the 20% that cause 80% of results).
9. Harness the power of simple formulas.
10. Be aware of context.

IV
HOW TO HAVE COMMON SENSE

Chapter 13

NO SPOONBENDING

We have now sunk to a depth at
which restatement of the obvious
is the first duty of intelligent men.

—George Orwell

A MAGICIAN NAMED URI GELLER RECEIVED widespread media attention in the United States in the 1970s. Geller claimed to be able to bend metal spoons using paranormal mind power. He appeared on many U.S. and European television programs to demonstrate. Critics showed that he used simple tricks. This did not stop Geller from making a living from the illusion that spoons can be bent with mind power.

Some people make a living selling the illusion that the life you want can be had without sacrifice and struggle. Common sense doesn't buy magical thinking.

Over one hundred million people in the United States go on a diet in any given year. Dieting is a growth business, despite and because of the fact that the customers fail to get the results they want.

There is copious spoonbending centered on the illusion of painless, convenient change: *Eat what you want and still lose weight!*

Spoons are not bent by magic. Losing weight is neither convenient nor painless. Even people who succeed tend to add the lost weight back in a year or two.

Every January many of us become powerfully infatuated with the idea of a new and improved version of ourselves: fit; organized; rich; and — above all — thin.

Infatuation knows nothing of common sense. We don't foresee, let alone prepare for, what Jung called "the laborious adaptations and manifold disappointments" that accompany any sort of significant personal progress. We buy soap instead: Spray 'n Change. The problem is not that this soap won't get us clean; the problem is that the sellers claim it will keep us clean forever. And they want $972 per bar.

What we spend is not surprising. America is a rich and optimistic nation. Most of us hope to be better than we are now. What *is* surprising is how poorly most of these products perform. Their goal is to overcome your resistance to buying, not your bad habit. Spoonbenders encourage passive consumption over creative suffering. They are false guides. They direct you away from where you need to go.

There are two types of spoonbenders in the self-help marketplace: Easy and Magic. Easy promises that you'll change with almost no effort, because of their unique product. Magic promises that you'll change via incredible feats of mind power, to which they have the secret.

Easy starts with this premise: *Do* better at this one thing (whitening your teeth, conditioning your hair, losing weight) and you will *be* better. (I've met a few skinny jerks with great hair and white teeth.)

Easy overpromises: This is going to be (pick one) effortless/convenient/cheap. Possibly, if your goal is controlling dandruff. Absolutely not for more profound changes, such as a mature long-term approach to diet and exercise.

Nevertheless, in one form or another, the siren cry of "eat what you want and still lose weight" echoes throughout the marketplace. The only way to do that, my friend, is to change what you want to eat. Simple. Not easy.

Magic also starts with a reasonable premise: *Be* better and you will *do* better. But then they get out the spoons.

As sociologist Micki McGee points out in *Self-Help, Inc.*, the people who sell Magic often take a mystical approach. Some borrow from the traditions of evangelical Christianity and use revival-style meetings to deliver their message and sell their merchandise. They replace snake handling with fire walking or some other vivid but irrelevant activity.

There is an exaggerated focus — like Uri Geller — on mind power. We are told that positive thinking and proper mental alignment will quickly cause improvement in externals such as bank accounts, advancement at work, and family relationships.

Yes, we know people can call forth latent courage to do more and be more. But Magic makes it sound so easy and so final. Like painless weight loss.

If that doesn't get you to open your wallet, Magic declares that the power is not within *us*, but out *there*. You grow your wealth, lose weight, get happier, and bend spoons by aligning yourself with the universe, which will provide you with abundant prosperity. Being broke is just a blockage of energy. Magic advises opening up your channel so money and consumer goods can flow through: "Prepare your wish list to the universe." Prepare for spoonbending.

Everything you want is out there awaiting delivery, if only you will provide the correct address. The "Laws of Attraction," like the laws of painless weight loss, are much more convenient than the work of real change. Magic says "This will be easy, this will not require sacrifices." Also not required: common sense.

Magic paints lovely visions of material and personal success. As with a lottery ticket, it is helpful to keep the long odds in mind.

Like Uri Geller's spoonbending, close inspection reveals the content of the message to be less compelling than the delivery. This is a new-age version of "eat what you want and still lose weight." So-called universal laws gain traction on our wallets through magical thinking, the absence of common sense.

Some Magic is pseudo-rational rather than mystical. As McGee points out, we get customized versions of the traditional life-as-journey metaphor: You are the CEO of your life; life is a work of art; life is like managing an investment portfolio. Conflicts come with win-win solutions, which can be found by drawing on one's emotional bank account.

Heroic feats of productivity are part of Magic. Not a moment will be lost. The apps, the hacks, the trading software, the notebooks, the juiced-up calendars and to-do lists online and off are indispensable implements for the superhuman parsing of every minute of every day.

I agree with Micki: This is another version of limitless mind power. Somehow there is limitless knowledge, time, and energy for self-discipline and industriousness. Count your spoons.

Not all the products offered by Easy and Magic are without value. But like that $972 bar of soap, they are overpriced and oversold. Despite initial appearances, Easy and Magic promote passive behavior, including passive consumption. Raspberry ketones!

Their nostrums are diversions from the more challenging work of real change. Real change begins with understanding the predictable weakness of human logic, and searching for the reasons why you can't or won't do better. That takes more than soap.

After Easy and Magic comes Perfect. Perfect confuses performance with results. It ignores the role of forces outside of our control, including randomness and luck. Perfect doesn't allow for human fallibility.

Perfect is a trap. Striving to be excellent is not. Excellence is from process and growth, not outcomes and opinions of others.

To be a perfect dieter requires a perfect diet and a perfect you. Not gonna happen. But dieting *can* make you better than you were. You *can* learn about yourself by paying attention to the process. You *can* become a better person, and a better dieter. A little *closer* to perfect.

Perhaps the self-improvement program you select will give you the tools you need to become better. Don't let that confuse you. The spade does not plant the garden. It is not the program that is changing you; *you* are changing you.

The quarterback hands the football to the halfback. Two guards pull from the offensive line and lead him around the end. The tight end blocks the linebacker on that side. Here comes the power sweep.

The Green Bay Packers, winners of the first two Super Bowls, ran the simple power sweep over and over: 28: left; 49: right.

Adapted by Vince Lombardi from the old single wing offense, the play was strategically mediocre. It was simple, and easy to recognize. Opposing defenses knew the Green Bay power sweep was coming at them several times a game. They just couldn't stop it.

The reason was execution. Due to constant repetition in practice and on the playing field, the Packers executed the play brilliantly. The Green Bay power sweep: a mediocre plan plus sound execution creates excellence.

Alternating days of Bikram Yoga, weight training, and swimming a mile is a brilliant plan for getting fit. It uses all the muscles, is interesting, lets you buy three different cool outfits, and is guaranteed to give anyone under seventy a great body. Just walking for thirty minutes every day: mediocre.

Which program do you think most of us will be more likely to stick to over the course of a year? Those Speedos won't get the job done from the closet.

We are going to make baby food from organic local vegetables; we are going to use only cloth diapers; we are going to iron those diapers; we are going to play classical music for baby every day; and we are going to employ only college graduates as babysitters. A brilliant plan for raising a healthy child. Fuhgeddaboudit.

We are going to keep our children reasonably clean and properly clothed and fed. We will read to them when we can, not scream at them when we are exhausted, and take them to the doctor when they get sick. We will do our best to let them know they are loved. That is a plan most parents can pull off. Hey baby, let's try *that*.

> *Young mouse: We will put a bell around the cat's*
> *neck, so we hear it coming!*
> *Old mouse: 'Tis well said, but who dares bell the cat?*

Physician Atul Gawande writes about the yawning gap between our nation's ability to develop breakthrough therapies for disease and our ability to make them effective. Huge advances are made in medicine. Brilliant plans are written for improving public health. What is overlooked by government, foundations, and academia is blocking and tackling, the boring — crucial — task of execution.

Our approach to health care resembles the flea flicker: an entertaining, elaborate, and unpredictable football play. Anything but the simple Green Bay power sweep. Result? We are way behind.

New discoveries and new ideas are vivid and inspiring. They fill us with enthusiasm. We forget to plan the work of making them work. We forget about the laborious adaptations and manifold disappointments of personal development. The bright idea is fascinating. Execution is boring, the opposite of Easy and Magic. But like Easy and Magic, bright ideas will not get us past Day Four.

FUNDAMENTALS of KEEPING YOUR SPOONS STRAIGHT

1. Don't confuse Easy and Magic with the work of real change.
2. To eat what you want and still lose weight, you have to change what you want.
3. Don't lead with your wallet.
4. Perfectionism is a means of avoiding change.
5. Sound execution is more important than a brilliant plan.

GUMPTIONWORK

Unbend
Your Spoon

You can also do this online:
www.gumptionade.com/unbend-my-spoon

1. I had a program (diet, investment, getting organized, parenting, et al.) that I hoped would help me reach an important goal.
   ☐ Yes ☐ No

   If yes, please proceed to number two below. If no, stop here and proceed to Chapter 14.

2. How much time did the program cost me?

   _____

3. How much money did the program cost me?

   _____

4. Did I believe any of the following promises:

I will:	*This will be:*
1. look younger	1. fast
2. get rich	2. painless
3. lose weight	3. convenient
4. be popular	4. easy
5. find love	5. free

   ☐ Yes ☐ No

GUMPTIONWORK

Did I get a poor return on my investment?
☐ Yes ☐ No

Was it a brilliant, exciting plan, rather than a simple, boring plan?
☐ Yes ☐ No

Did I give up when things didn't go as I hoped?
☐ Yes ☐ No

Fool me once, shame on them. Fool me twice, shame on me.
☐ Yes ☐ No

Chapter 14

KNOW YOUR MIND

Our cerebral consciousness is
like an actor who has forgotten
that he is playing a role.

C. G. JUNG

I SET OFF FOR COSTCO ON SATURDAY MORN-
ing. When I hit the first red light, I could not remember
a thing about the previous four miles. My car had been
driven by a section of my mind operating independently. How?

Because my brain has an autopilot that can engage when
I drive familiar routes, leaving me free to think about money
and sex.

I am a thirty-four-year-old man at a family Thanksgiving in
Memphis. I find myself remembering my second-grade class-
room at P.S. 6 in New York. That was 1963. I feel the same
vague sense of discomfort that I felt then. Why?

Because my little nephew on the floor behind me has
opened up a glue stick. The smell unearths long-forgotten
feelings from a sub-basement in my head. What else is down
there in the dark?

It is mid-April of my senior year at Kenyon College. I have
not been to German class all semester. The final exam is
approaching. I will not graduate if I flunk this class. I want to
get there and try to catch up, but I don't know when or where
the class meets. What is this?

It's my standard anxiety dream. In one variation, I am not
wearing pants. When I wake up, I'm always relieved to remember that I have graduated. Then I usually remember something
coming up, for which I'm not yet prepared.

What's the force behind all this activity?

Understanding how your mind works — and doesn't — strengthens common sense. That's important: To do what needs to be
done, you have to choose the right *what*. That requires common sense.

Let's start by admitting that much human decision making
is not rational. People are *not* logical. People are *psycho*-logical.
Important choices are driven by emotion.

You are largely unaware of what goes on between your ears.
That makes you normal.

Leaving out consideration of an eternal soul, there are two
parts to you: a body and a mind. Beyond your body is a vast
external space: city, nation, planet, and universe. You *know*
only an infinitesimal part of that space. Behind your conscious mind is a vast *internal* space; your *un*conscious mind.
It's bigger.

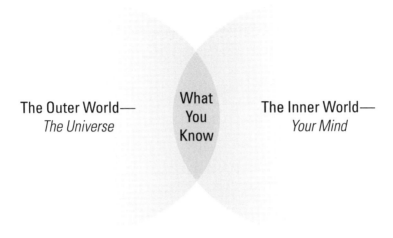

The Outer World—   What   The Inner World—
The Universe   You   *Your Mind*
                          Know

"What You Know" Is the Small Overlap of Two Large Worlds

The thoughts of your conscious mind are *visible* reference points: I hate the Yankees…I love french fries…I'm too hot… my left foot itches…here's Butch, my neighbor's Rottweiler. Butch is not a danger to me.

The thoughts of your *un*conscious mind are your *invisible* reference points. They have great power. This is not news. As Leonard Mlodinow notes in *Subliminal*, philosophers and scientists since Plato have recognized there is much more to our behavior than can be explained by visible, direct causes.

Do you ever look back and wonder why on earth you would say such a thing…buy that…eat so much…drink so much… choose someone so unsuitable? And why on earth you would do it again? You can't see your invisible reference points. But you *can* see their footprints.

> *The most decisive qualities in a person are often*
> *unconscious and can be perceived only by others, or*
> *have to be laboriously discovered with outside help.*
>
> C. G. Jung

Your brain is adapted for pre-historic life on the African savannah. You have inherited ways of thinking and acting from Your Hairy Ancestor that don't work when you're looking at a carton of French vanilla ice cream or stuck in traffic on the George Washington Bridge.

You have also inherited ways of thinking and acting from The Child You Were. These include curiosity, playfulness, and poor impulse control. That child is a force of things in your marriage, your relationships with your children, your work life. Like Your Hairy Ancestor, The Child You Were is always with you. And the kid in short pants has opinions.

Mlodinow points out you have the brain Your Hairy Ancestor developed to survive. Then as now, living required processing a huge amount of external information while carrying out a huge amount of internal activity.

Part of your unconscious mind controls your vital behind-the-scenes functions, such as digestion, breathing, and vision. These are not trivial demands. About a third of your brain is devoted to vision.

Your unconscious mind also controls some external activities — as when you drive for miles with no memory of having done so. There's a lot going on there. In the dark.

The clamorous reed warbler nests, flies, and sings despite being unknown to you. If you want to be a better bird watcher, you must increase your knowledge of the world of birds. That world includes Asian songbirds.

So also for your inner world. The fact that you are unaware of most of your thoughts doesn't mean they aren't there. If you want to get more common sense — make better choices — you must increase your knowledge of the world inside your head.

It's not easy to think about your own thinking. Your Hairy Ancestor was better at reacting than reflecting. Helpful when the driver ahead of you stops suddenly and your foot automatically hits the brake.

Less helpful if he flips you off. Instead of seeing an idiot, your brain sees a threat and — without consulting you — activates your fight-or-flight response. A flood of adrenaline and cortisol increases your heart rate, dilates your pupils, and focuses your vision. Useful if you're being stalked by a saber-toothed tiger. Not so much during rush hour on that bridge in New Jersey.

My unconscious mind drives my two-ton, five-speed automobile. It instantly retrieves a memory from 1963. It wakes me in a sweat over an exam that I do not have to take. What else can my unconscious do?

> *I do not love thee, Dr. Fell.*
> *The reason why, I cannot tell;*
> *But this I know, and know full well,*
> *I do not love thee, Dr. Fell.*
> Tom Brown

My unconscious can and will project some of its contents onto other people.

Some of these projections are obvious and temporary. Tom was on his way to make a sales presentation to the California Public Employees' Retirement System (CalPERS). He was going to present his company's WBT Investment Fund — whiskey, bullets, and tobacco — as a diversification opportunity. It him took a year to get this meeting.

But Tom's flight to Sacramento left without him. First, he got a late start that morning. Then a tanker truck spilled guacamole on the Santa Monica Freeway, forcing him onto city streets.

The line to get through security at LAX was monstrous. Tom was more than a little tense as he finally approached his gate at a jog. The door to the clearly visible airplane had just closed, per regulations, fifteen minutes before takeoff.

The gate agent would not unlock the door. Tom realized he was going to miss his big meeting. He exploded, shouting abuse at her and her airline before storming off.

Then he calmed down. Then he mustered a little courage and sought out that gate agent and asked forgiveness. He had projected his anger and fear onto her. His fear of a loss of income. His anger at himself for leaving everything until the last minute, as usual.

CalPERS let him make his presentation the following week, by the way. They then declined the opportunity to invest public pension assets in bullets and tobacco, despite the obvious financial advantages.

If you allow what you know about a person to influence what you don't, you are subject to the force of a projection called the halo effect.

Major league baseball umpires expand the strike zone for veteran pitchers.

Teachers told that certain of their students had scored high on I.Q. testing — they had actually made average scores — later rated these students as more curious and interested than average students. They received higher grades as well.

Most of us believe physically attractive people are more likely to be better parents, have better marriages, and be generally happier than people with average looks. They are not. Due to the halo effect, however, they *are* more likely to get elected to public office.

History is full of examples of critics praising the mediocre work of successful artists while brilliant work from unknowns is ignored. Vincent van Gogh sold only one painting in his lifetime, *Red Vineyard at Arles* — now worth more at auction than the gross national product of Burundi — and that was to his friend's sister.

Something good *can* come out of Nazareth, but most people won't notice.

The new love of your life is really the most attractive, enchanting, brilliant person you have ever met and nothing would be better than to spend the rest of your life with him. The fact that he bears an uncanny resemblance to your charismatic father — an irresponsible bon vivant — escapes you. After many months and many disappointments, you come to your senses. Your conscious mind wonders what on earth you were thinking. Later, you'll fall for another guy like that. And another. Until you're smart enough or fed up enough to get to the root of your fixation. To see the heretofore invisible reference point you project onto charming man-boys. Simple. Not easy.

It is a given among marriage counselors that you can and will project your feelings about one of your parents onto your spouse. My own actions reveal a preference that the role of Bob's Wife be filled by a strong and independent woman. This is due in great measure to the personality of my strong, independent, and opinionated mother. She was a real handful and so is my wife. And the two before her.

The child I was when my beloved mother dominated the scene lives on through reference points in my unconscious that are as vital as the day they were laid down. They pull me back to early childhood, when I was — from time to time — resentful and even fearful of my mother's power over me.

Under duress, I will project these fears and resentments onto Bob's Wife. To be a good enough husband, I have to manually override this psycho-logic. Simple. Not easy.

For decades I was under the illusion I was free to choose. I was unaware of the force behind my attraction to a certain kind

of woman — and my resentment. Therapy helped me see that
I was an actor, playing a role written and directed by a part of
my mind standing offstage. My unconscious drove me as eas-
ily as it drives my Honda. Just much, much further.

What else can it do?

> *Contempt is the weapon of the weak, a defense*
> *against one's own despised and unwanted feelings.*
> ALICE MILLER

I once worked with someone who was vocal about his disdain for gay men. As it happens, he was a very smart dresser
and somewhat effeminate. Seemed a good fellow to me.

It also seemed to me, armchair psychologist, that his contempt was driven by his unconscious fear that *he* was gay. I
don't know if he was or not, but if we had been friends I would
have bestowed my opinion on him. (Why don't I have more
friends?)

The traits people dislike in others are often traits they dislike in themselves. I am contemptuous of people who have to
be the center of attention. [*Author pauses to clear throat*] But
now I know why. Now I can set aside my reflexive attitude —
my psycho-logic — when I meet a person who is like me in
that way.

Racial, ethnic, and religious groups carry invisible reference points. Mass projections of fear, anger and insecurity can
erupt, with dire consequences. Historians see a clear correlation between low cotton prices and the lynching of blacks in
the South during the early twentieth century.

What was the force of that thing? In the era before government farm supports and social welfare programs, low cotton prices caused widespread poverty — and widespread *fear* of poverty — in the cotton-growing states.

Contempt is a weapon of the weak. The force at work was the projection of fear and anger onto a scapegoat group by economically endangered whites. This was aided and abetted by elected officials whose short-term political interests were an incentive to ignore laws against kidnapping and murder.

Whole nations can be driven by psycho-logic. The Nazi genocide was caused in part by a mass projection onto Jews of the anger, humiliation, and fear felt during the economic and social upheavals that followed Germany's defeat in World War I.

Magnifying the force of this projection was the time-honored status of Jews as outsiders. The Germans needed a scapegoat. As usual, there was also an economic incentive. Some German Jews owned businesses and other property that could be stolen by the government when they were arrested.

Contempt is a weapon of the weak. Be strong. Look for the cause of your need to find a scapegoat.

Your mind has two parts. "The Me I Know" stands in the light. "The Me I Don't" is in the dark. To have more common sense — to have more gumption — drag as much you can into the light. Study your reference points. Look for footprints left by shadows. Think about your thinking. This is what makes you an adult.

But it's still okay to hate the Yankees. Or at least to hate the things the Yankees *do*.

FUNDAMENTALS of YOUR MIND

1. There is logic and then there is psycho-logic.
2. Your mind consists of two parts. The small part contains the thoughts and feelings you know about. The big part contains the ones you don't.
3. Invisible reference points manifest themselves in the behaviors you engage in without understanding why.
4. Many of these reference points are inherited from Your Hairy Ancestor or The Child You Were.
5. People unknowingly project their feelings onto others.
6. To increase common sense, move more of your key reference points into consciousness.

GUMPTIONWORK

A Short Guide to Reference Points

You can do this better online:
www.gumptionade.com/reference-points

Review the examples provided and write in examples of your own invisible reference points, if you please.

FOOTPRINT	VISIBLE REFERENCE POINT	INVISIBLE REFERENCE POINT
Fear of spiders	You think spiders are creepy.	Instinctive avoidance behavior toward poisonous creatures
Choice of spouse	You're in love.	Similarity to a parent
Racial prejudice	How stupid, bad, and/or different those people are.	Tribal instinct, fear
Obsessive neatness	Things should be in their place.	Anxiety
Anorexia	You're so fat.	Feelings of lack of control
Promiscuity	You need to have sex with many partners.	You need intense experiences to feel anything.
Obesity	You can't control your eating habits.	Your Hairy Ancestor's famine survival instincts

GUMPTIONWORK

FOOTPRINT	VISIBLE REFERENCE POINT	INVISIBLE REFERENCE POINT
Drug use	You like being high.	You prefer not to deal with life as an adult.
Workaholic behavior	You want to be rich and famous.	You have to achieve to feel worthy.
Reader's Choice	Reader's Choice	Reader's Choice
Reader's Choice	Reader's Choice	Reader's Choice
Reader's Choice	Reader's Choice	Reader's Choice
Reader's Choice	Reader's Choice	Reader's Choice
Reader's Choice	Reader's Choice	Reader's Choice
Reader's Choice	Reader's Choice	Reader's Choice
Reader's Choice	Reader's Choice	Reader's Choice
Reader's Choice	Reader's Choice	Reader's Choice

Chapter 15

BE LESS WRONG

Sometimes you feel like a nut,
sometimes you don't.

Leon Carr

ET ME PUT YOU IN AN EXPERIMENT CON-
ducted by Nobel Prize-winning psychologists Daniel
Kahneman and Amos Tversky: You and several other
people are sitting in a room. At the front of the room is a num-
bered game wheel, the kind you see at a fair. A woman spins
it. The wheel is rigged to stop on the number sixty-five. You
are not told this.

It stops on sixty-five. The woman asks everyone to write
down that number. She then asks you to answer a few questions, including this one: What percentage of UN member
states are African?

The answer that you and the others give averages out to
forty-five percent. The average answer of a different group of
people, who saw the wheel land on the number ten, was much
lower: twenty-five percent.

A Way to Be Wrong Known as Anchoring

Number the game wheel stopped on	Estimate of UN member states that are African
65	45%
10	25%

Like most of us, you have a weakness for anchoring. You can be influenced by an irrelevant number on a game wheel. Your logic about African states and the UN is psycho-logic.

Disinterested speculation about the UN is one thing, but would anchoring ever affect an important personal decision? Yes. A woman whose maiden name is Brown is more likely to marry another Brown than a Smith or a Jones, despite the fact that there are more Smiths and Joneses out there. People are anchored to their own name.

It's not common sense to be influenced by irrelevant reference points. It's just normal.

Your brain does a lot of work without asking your permission. It's good that you don't forget to breathe. But anchoring and other glitches in your automatic thinking weaken your common sense. Many of them can be organized into four categories:

The Four Pillars of Wrongness

1. Loss Aversion
2. Hindsight Bias
3. Myopic Forecasting
4. The Illusion of Memory

1. LOSS AVERSION

The hunter makes a hole in a coconut. Bigger than Monkey's hand, smaller than Monkey's fist. The hunter fills the coconut halfway with rice — Monkey's favorite food — and stakes it tight to the ground. Monkey happens by, reaches into the coconut, and grabs a fistful of rice. Now Monkey is stuck. Now the hunter returns. Will Monkey drop the rice and escape? Maybe not. Maybe Monkey wants rice too much.

Monkey is in danger of dying from loss aversion. She bears risk of capture to avoid the pain of losing a fistful of rice. She is caught by her thinking before she is caught by the hunter.

I worked at an advertising agency that was in the finals of a competition for the business of a large restaurant franchise group. Winning this account would be a great triumph. We really wanted it.

At the cost of seven hundred dollars, we designed and produced about three dozen blue cardboard signs to be held up at various times during our pitch. Each sign had a quote from consumer research we had done. This would show how smart we were, and how well we understood the hamburger business.

It became clear in rehearsal that the blue signs did not work. They distracted attention from the focus of our remarks, which had changed after the signs were made.

I suggested that we ditch the blue signs but was overruled by a more senior executive on the pitch. They were his idea. He had approved the seven-hundred-dollar expense.

We used the blue signs. Our presentation was disjointed. We did not win the McDonald's account.

Senior man chased seven hundred dollars down a rabbit hole and took us with him. He lost sight of the multimillion-dollar opportunity. For which we had waited five years. What invisible force made him more interested in using the blue signs than in making the best possible pitch?

Loss aversion: His unconscious embraced the risk of a poor presentation to avoid the pain of regret over a failed idea and the loss of seven hundred dollars. Wrongness.

Imagine you and Bill Gates are having a few cold ones at Chili's. He puts five one hundred dollar bills on the bar and offers you this choice: "Take this five hundred dollars or flip a coin. If it lands on heads, I'll pay you one thousand dollars. Tails you get nothing."

As most people would, you choose the sure five hundred. Thanks, Bill.

Gates orders a cheeseburger, then lays out five more Benjamins. "You now have one thousand dollars. But you must choose," he says. "Will you lose five hundred of it guaranteed, or flip the coin and take a fifty percent chance of losing the entire one thousand dollars."

As most people would, you flip the coin and accept the risk of losing one thousand dollars to avoid a sure loss of five hundred dollars.

Bill then points out how changeable you are: First you wanted a guaranteed five hundred dollars. Then you rejected a guaranteed five hundred.

If you are normal, you will take risks to avoid a loss that you would not take for an equivalent or even bigger gain. If you are normal, loss aversion can turn your money logic into psycho-logic. Wrongness.

Dan and Amos both want to see their Jumbos play the Bombers—bitter rivals   tonight. They both live in the same suburb, about an hour's drive from the Fudge Forum, home of the Jumbos. Dan bought his ninety-five-dollar ticket to the game this morning. Amos bought his a few months ago.

It starts to snow around 4:00 p.m. It is soon obvious there will be dangerous weather tonight. The Jumbos and the Bombers will play the game, but Dan and Amos face the disappointment of missing it. Which of them is more likely to risk the drive? That is to say, which of them is more likely to be wrong?

Having bought his ticket this morning, Dan will chase his ninety-five dollars through a blizzard, notwithstanding the fact that on any other weeknight, ninety-five dollars would not be enough to get him to drive all the way downtown and back in a light drizzle.

Dan fails to stop and ask himself two simple questions: "Would I drive through a blizzard if I had been given this ticket?" He would not. "Then why would I do it now?" After all, a ticket is a ticket, regardless of where it came from.

That is so logical. People are *so* psycho-logical.

Dan starts toward downtown and ends up being dropped off at home at 4:00 a.m. by the state police, his car abandoned on the highway, not having gotten within ten miles of the game.

The force of loss aversion made Dan's *imagined* pain of regret loom large in his unconscious mind. He accepted great risk to avoid this loss. Wrongness. Where was his common sense? Where was his gumption? Where, Monkey, where?

In December 1965, Frankie Valli and the Four Seasons reached number three on the Billboard chart with "Let's Hang On (To What We've Got)." This is a cry that originates deep in the human unconscious.

Loss aversion was — and is — a subset of death aversion. To stay alive, Your Hairy Ancestor had to survive the process of getting food and shelter. Loss of food threatened death by starvation. Loss of shelter threatened death by exposure.

Movement invited attack by other survivors, including saber-toothed tigers and fellow proto-humans. Replacing lost necessities was uncertain at best and fatal at worst.

The threat of loss received a more powerful response than the opportunity for gain among those individuals who survived long enough to *be* your ancestor.

Reference points laid down a million years ago influence your intuitive response to modern threats, including threats that are more symbolic than actual. Such as the loss of a ninety-five-dollar Jumbos ticket. Such as the loss of seven hundred dollars' worth of blue signs. Not life or death matters, but you would think so by what happened.

Why don't you have more common sense? Why can't you tell the difference between real and symbolic threats? Why this wrongness? Because, as Leonard Mlodinow neatly put it, evolution designed your brain for survival, not self-awareness.

2. HINDSIGHT BIAS

What are the odds that I would find myself in March of 2015 sitting at a desk in Memphis, Tennessee? The path from New Haven, Connecticut, where I was born, is strewn with happenstance and coincidence.

One example: The brother of a college roommate happened to work at Procter & Gamble. Because he visited and told me about his job, I applied there and ended up living in Cincinnati. Then I was transferred. It just so happened that a P&G subsidiary in Memphis needed someone with my experience.

Completely unremarkable. It seems so inevitable now. But how predictable was this outcome on July 19, 1956, the day I was born?

It is unlikely that I would be anywhere at all. What were the odds of my parents, born in different cities, meeting and producing any offspring together, let alone me?

My father had to be born, survive his army service in World War II, and go to college, for which the GI Bill had to pass Congress in 1944. He had to take a certain freshman biology class and receive an invitation by his professor for Sunday dinner, where he met my mother. And they had to get along.

And by the way, all of the ancestors of both my parents had to survive childhood, successfully reproduce, and raise at least one child that did the same.

The odds here are less than one in several trillion. Winning the Mega Millions is a sure thing in comparison. But I'm sitting here in Memphis, drinking coffee, and smoking big cigars.

Your mind projects wrongness on the world via hindsight bias, the sense that what happened was bound to happen. Randomness docs not look random. You overlook the decisive role of chance. Certainty is an illusion. And this illusion can cover the rocks while you sail right onto them. Wrongness.

Bill Belichick is a lucky so-and so. Have you seen his girlfriend? His New England Patriots' brilliant success over the last dozen years seems so inevitable now: the future Hall of Fame quarterback; the genius coach; the great organization. How else could it have turned out?

Differently. Their first two Super Bowls were won by field goals of more than forty yards, kicked in the last ten seconds of each game. The Patriots' most recent title came when their opponent pulled defeat out of the jaws of victory. In their four Super Bowl wins, the Patriots' average margin of victory was just three points.

By comparison, the Green Bay Packers outscored their first two Super Bowl opponents by an average of twenty-two points, more than *seven* field goals' worth of margin.

The Patriots' image is improved by hindsight bias. We remember the past imperfectly. We forget the parts that don't fit the narrative we have now. We remember the skill but forget the luck. Wrongness.

Imagine all the people in the world are sitting in one room. Each holds a coin. They all stand up and begin flipping their coins. They sit down when it comes up tails. The last person standing will have seen their coin come up heads thirty-two times in a row.

There's no skill involved. It's a function of base size: We started with seven billion coin flips. But our winner could be forgiven if she thought she were something special. She is not. She is no more likely than you are to get heads next time. (This concept applies handsomely to high-flying mutual funds, by the way.)

When you see a successful person, you are often looking at the winner of an extended series of coin tosses. Probably smart and hardworking, since those characteristics dramatically leverage the value of luck. A coin-toss winner nonetheless. Hindsight bias obscures the role of chance in their achievement. As Paul Getty said, the secret to success is to get up early, work hard, and strike oil.

Would milkshake mixer salesman Ray Kroc have sold billions of hamburgers if the owners of a drive-in restaurant — the McDonald brothers — had not astounded him by purchasing eight of his Prince Castle five-spindle Multimixers? Would George W. Bush have been president if he had been born George W. Guànmù? Do you want fries with that?

It seems so certain now, but what were the odds that your friend Bill Gates would become the richest man in the world? Gates is brilliant, hardworking, and visionary. He is also lucky. Here are two examples: In 1968, when Gates was in the eighth grade, the Lakeside School Mothers' Club invested the proceeds from a rummage sale into a computer terminal and a block of time on a mainframe computer in downtown Seattle.

This decision dramatically increased the possibility that a kid at Lakeside Middle School could learn computer programming. Had the mothers' club bought the sorely needed movie projector instead, Bill Gates might have ended up a lawyer like his father.

A few years later, fledgling Microsoft was working on a programming language for IBM's first PC. As it happened, IBM was unable to purchase an operating system for the PC from Digital Research, the likeliest vendor. IBM asked Gates if Microsoft could help.

Although Microsoft did not have an operating system, he said they could (you have to take your luck). They bought one from Seattle Computer Products, tweaked it for the PC, and sold it to IBM for fifty thousand dollars. Microsoft kept the rights.

The shrewdness that Gates displayed dramatically increased the positive effects of his good luck. But you still could not have predicted Microsoft's extraordinary success the day before IBM said yes. Bill Gates won more than his share of coin flips along the way.

Hindsight bias is wrongness that distorts the past. Because common sense learns from the past, hindsight bias is wrongness that weakens common sense. When you look back, don't forget: things didn't have to turn out this way.

3. Myopic Forecasting

Humans are also nearsighted when they look ahead. Our predictions are influenced by how we feel when we make them. We unconsciously project what we *want* to happen, or *fear* will happen, onto what is *likely* to happen. Statistics — facts — about dieting, marriage, exercise, starting a business, motorcycle riding, and other activities may be sobering or they may be encouraging. But when people decide what to do, they pay more attention to how they feel.

Even if it's just feeling hungry. In *Thinking Fast and Slow*, Kahneman cites a study showing that judges paroled signifi cantly fewer prisoners in the hour before lunch compared to the rest of the day.

Any dieter will testify that hunger makes you pessimistic. But optimism can also impair common sense. Feeling good about your new diet doesn't mean you'll lose the weight...That stock *can* miss...He may *not* be the one for you...She can stop at one drink, but probably *won't*...Please tell me *how* we will finish by the deadline...What makes *this* time different?

As with other projections, groups as well as individuals can be fooled, in this case by optimistic reference points.

The Government Accountability Office recently testified that the Pentagon's costliest program, the F-35 fighter jet, is already $1 billion over budget. This is on top of $373 million for correcting deficiencies discovered in development testing. The GAO also testified that the F-35 has an unreliable design and an inefficient manufacturing process.

The Defense Department official responsible for acquisition says that the budget for the project had been based on "unfounded optimism." This is the same air force that paid $640 each for toilet seats. That's about as optimistic as you can get about a commode.

The average cost overrun on defense acquisition contracts is 40 percent. Why would anyone approach the budget for a new class of fighter aircraft with anything other than profound skepticism? Wrongness.

In 1985, Boston city officials optimistically projected that the Big Dig highway construction project would cost about $6 billion. The final bill was $22 billion. After construction was complete, the Boston Globe reported, "Ultimately, many motorists going to and from the suburbs are spending more time stuck in traffic rather than less." There have also been significant quality problems.

The Sydney Opera house opened ten years behind schedule and 1,300 percent over budget. And the original plan was scaled back significantly along the way.

> It is extremely difficult to see how five years from now
> we could be looking back and observing a historical
> 5-year growth rate of, say, less than 5%. That should
> be more than adequate to support the continued good
> credit performance of sub-prime mortgage pools.
>
> "HOUSING OUTLOOK," J.P. MORGAN RESEARCH, JUNE 17, 2005

This optimistic and incorrect prediction was made less than a year before the air started coming out of the U.S. housing bubble, triggering the financial debacle that caused a severe worldwide recession.

But J.P. Morgan sold a lot of bonds backed by subprime mortgage pools before everything went pear-shaped. The bank later paid a $13 billion fine to get the Justice Department to drop its civil suit over those sales. Thirteen billion. With a b. The price of myopia. Wrongness.

What made the men and women at Clairol bet their careers and their company's money on Touch of Yogurt shampoo? Was their optimism influenced by loss aversion? Did they embrace risk to recover earlier losses from Look of Buttermilk?

Plenty of myopic forecasts have ended up on the big screen:

1. *Cleopatra* — budgeted at two million 1963 dollars but costing forty-four million — forced Twentieth Century Fox to close for several months.
2. *Waterworld*, starring then red-hot Kevin Costner, was the most expensive film ever made at the time. It not only bombed at the box office, but cost 175 percent of its gigantic initial budget.
3. United Artists' fiscal disaster *Heaven's Gate* got so far behind schedule that several of the musicians required to be on location in Montana ended up living there.

Success is easy and pleasant to imagine. The many ways that things can and do fall apart are not.

Sometimes we aren't exactly fooled. Information that challenges our livelihood or our self-image will be overlooked. Defense suppliers are happy to go along with Pentagon forecasts, because the overages increase their profits. Boston concrete companies did not challenge the optimistic Big Dig forecast. If pressed, they might have said that any unforeseen problems could be solved by more concrete.

You love your plan to lose forty pounds on the Raspberry Ketone diet. Painless weight loss! Right now you are not interested in facts about sound dieting practices, the crucial role of exercise, or what you could learn from your previous dieting failures. You predict you will reach your ideal weight without suffering for it. I predict there will be laborious adaptations and manifold disappointments. I predict your beautiful plan will end up touched by yogurt. By wrongness.

Be on guard for myopic forecasting. Be less wrong. Use common sense when looking into the future, so you have gumption on Day Four.

4. The Illusion of Memory

Tommie is in an auditorium full of people. A man in an expensive suit is giving a lecture on investing. Tommie is thinking about lunch, about the disagreement she had with her husband this morning, and about the ink stain on her sleeve.

Suddenly a cowboy bursts through the back door of the auditorium and runs to the stage, pursued by a clown holding a pie. The cowboy and the clown stop there. They argue and the clown flings the pie, missing the cowboy but hitting the speaker. The clown runs back down the aisle and out the back door, closely followed by the cowboy. Now *that* is something Tommie is never going to forget.

Tommie is then told this was a staged event and immediately quizzed on what she saw. Among other things, she recalls that the cowboy wore a Stetson (typical of cowboys). He was in fact bareheaded. She gets the clown suit all wrong. She omits or unknowingly fabricates other important details. The accuracy of her clear, vivid, and *recent* memory is surprisingly poor.

To make a point about the problem with memory, I just put Tommie in my update of a late-nineteenth-century psychology experiment, described by Mlodinow in *Subliminal*.

It doesn't get any better with less vivid occurrences. In his book *Memory*, Ian Hunter cites a secretly recorded meeting of the Cambridge psychological society. Participants were tested on their memory of the meeting after two weeks. They had forgotten about 90 percent of what was discussed. Half the discussion they *did* recall never occurred. Wrongness.

Your brain does not store memories like a filing cabinet, a scrapbook, or a hard drive. A memory doesn't fade evenly over time like a photograph.

A memory more closely resembles a batch of cookies you repeatedly make in your head. The recipe is unwritten, one of thousands you know. Instead of ingredients, mixing procedures, cooking times and temperatures, there are the people involved, their actions and attitudes, the place, what you did, and what you felt.

People and their behaviors dominate memories the way the chocolate chips dominate the cookie recipe. Actions, traits, and *inferred* motives of the people involved stay vivid as other ingredients fade from memory.

Situational factors such as time pressure, weather, and noise are baking soda: crucial, but easy to forget.

You know there are chocolate chips in the mix, and you know that an oven is required. But you misremember proportions and forget or fabricate other ingredients.

You make the recipe as often as you remember the event. It gradually stabilizes into something predictable but far removed from the original. Your memory serves up something much smoother than the bumpy, irregular, and complicated chocolate chip cookies that were baked at the time. But you believe you have the original recipe. You are under the illusion that your memory is completely accurate. Wrongness.

We think we remember facts, but instead we construct artifacts. We believe we largely understand the past. We largely do not.

Suffering under this illusion, we tend to overestimate how predictable the future will be. This is not common sense. This is not gumption.

If you are going to find a way to do the thing that needs to be done, when it needs to be done, you'll have to learn how to be less wrong. Loss aversion, hindsight bias, myopic forecasting, and the illusion of memory weaken your common sense. Be on guard as you make decisions and you will have more gumption.

There is, by the way, another dangerous wrongness, one that needs no further explanation. It is the illusion that you don't have to wrestle with this frustrating, random, beautiful world to make a life worth living. It is the wrongness of Spray 'n Change.

FUNDAMENTALS
of WRONGNESS

1. Your judgment can be profoundly influenced by irrelevant reference points.
2. Loss aversion affects your decision making.
3. You underestimate the role of luck and randomness in the outcome of events.
4. Your predictions about the future are influenced by your mood.
5. Your memory of past events can be misleading.

GUMPTIONWORK
How to Be
Less Wrong
A Checklist for Making Better Decisions

You can do this better online:
www.gumptionade.com/less-wrong-decisions

Increase your common sense by reviewing the following list:

1. Create a simple formula for making a big decision. What are the three to five key points? Assign a certain weight to each point, according to its importance. For example, when I choose a car, I put forty percent of the weight of my decision on mechanical reliability; forty percent on price; twenty percent on good mileage. You might have a different system for weighing what matters most to you. Make sure that your total adds up to one hundred percent.

2. Guard against motivated reasoning. Be less of a lawyer (starting with a conclusion — "I can afford that BMW" — and finding evidence to support it) and more of a scientist (following facts *to* a conclusion — "All told, the BMW will cost me nine hundred and seventy dollars a month to own and operate. Can I afford that?").

3. Stop and consider why your thinking may be wrong. One way to do this is to hold a pre-mortem: "If this turns out badly, what would be the three most likely reasons why?"

   a. _____

   b. _____

   c. _____

GUMPTIONWORK

4. Answer this: "If someone else were in this situation, how would I advise them?"

_____

_____

5. Stop and ask yourself:

   a. Am I pursuing sunk costs? *(Chasing lost money and/or time — loss aversion)*
      ☐ Yes ☐ No
   Please explain: _____

   _____

   b. Am I embracing too much risk to prevent a loss? *(Also loss aversion)*
      ☐ Yes ☐ No
   Please explain: _____

   _____

   c. Am I assuming a best case scenario for the results of my decision? *(Myopic forecasting)*
      ☐ Yes ☐ No

   d. If yes, what is a more balanced forecast?

   _____

   _____

   e. Am I considering the impact of randomness and luck? *(The illusion of predictability)*
      ☐ Yes ☐ No

6. If you want to get a usable poll reading, aggregate the ten most recent polls on the topic.

FUNDAMENTALS of
COMMON SENSE

1. Do not confuse Easy and Magic with the real work of positive change.
2. A mediocre plan with sound execution always beats a brilliant plan with mediocre execution.
3. The brain Your Hairy Ancestor bequeathed you was designed for survival, not self-reflection.
4. You are often psycho-logical instead of logical.
5. Many of your personal reference points are emotional, not rational.
6. Many of your personal reference points are invisible to you (but sometimes obvious to others).
7. Consider the incentives of others when evaluating what they want you to do. These others include The Child You Were.
8. Monitor the feelings you project onto others. They are footprints you can track back to feelings about yourself of which you are unaware.
9. You will take greater risk to avoid losses than to achieve gains.
10. Your predictions of the future are over-influenced by your present mood.
11. Luck and randomness play a larger role in your life than you know.

Why Common Sense
<u>Is</u> Not Common

Every man carries with him the
world in which he must live.

F. Marion Crawford

There are two reasons why you sometimes act without common sense. They aren't your fault, but—since you are an adult—you are responsible for the consequences. They are:

Kryptonite to Common Sense

1. the power of your unconscious thoughts and feelings
2. the predictable shortcomings of human judgment and decision making

Your adult mind is fine-tuned for two worlds that no longer exist: the collective world of Your Hairy Ancestor and the individual world of The Child You Were. Actually, these worlds *do* exist. They exist in your mind, in the dark.

You are a ship piloted by three captains. You, the adult, are visible at the helm. Your Hairy Ancestor and The Child You Were have their invisible hands next to yours on the wheel. When you are not paying close attention (i.e., most of the

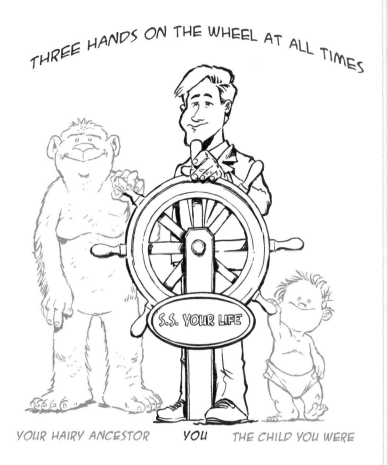

THREE HANDS ON THE WHEEL AT ALL TIMES

S.S. YOUR LIFE

YOUR HAIRY ANCESTOR   YOU   THE CHILD YOU WERE

time), they steer the ship. Often they steer it well. Sometimes they steer the ship onto the rocks. Sometimes your logic is psycho-logic.

If you marry, then there are six captains on the bridge. This is called a committee.

V

HOW TO GO FROM HERE

Chapter 16

CHOOSE

But the Hebrew word, the word timshel—
"Thou mayest"—that gives a choice. It might
be the most important word in the world. That
says the way is open. That throws it right
back on a man. For if "Thou mayest"—it
is also true that "Thou mayest not."

JOHN STEINBECK, EAST OF EDEN

LLEN WHEELIS WROTE ABOUT A CONCEN-
tration camp inmate pondering whether to struggle
on the way to the gas chamber and be shot for resisting, or to wait and be executed a few minutes later. History will
record only the constraints he was under and consider him a
victim. Wheelis argues that—even in this situation—the prisoner can make a choice: "For if he knows the constraint and
nothing else, if he thinks 'Nothing is possible,' then he is living his necessity; but if perceiving the constraint, he turns from

it to a choice between two possible courses of action, then —
however he choose — he is living his freedom."

If the prisoner can choose to live his freedom at *that*
moment, then surely we can in our lives. But do we?

You can choose to live your freedom, to become more
than you are now, or you can live your necessities, stand pat,
or even shrink. Your character is defined by the choices you
make. The quality of your life is defined by the quality of
your character.

As Huxley said, "Perhaps the most valuable result of all
education is the ability to make yourself do the thing you
have to do, when it ought to be done, whether you like it or
not." *What has to be done is to choose better.* That requires
courage, resourcefulness, and common sense. Choosing better requires gumption.

Randomness will be a force of things in your life. So will
your family and friends, your employer, your culture, Your
Hairy Ancestor, and The Child You Were. Regardless of the
gifts they give and the constraints they apply, you will always
have choices. Once in a while, on the important things,
choosing well invites discomfort and requires courage.

You may or may not be courageous when the time comes.
The greater danger, though, is that you will be blind to the
choice in front of you. A powerful force of things — the force
of habit — may disguise your choice as no choice, a forgone
conclusion, out of your control. To overcome this danger you
have to be resourceful enough to frame your decisions so you
can *see* the important choice. Don't guess. Know.

One morning in June of 2004 I woke up and finally saw what had been coming for years: The life I wanted — the life I knew — had ceased to be. I was no longer a young man, a family man, a member of the upper middle class, and a whip-smart entrepreneur. The family that meant so much to me was gone. The business success my ego needed so desperately had slipped from my grasp.

I dropped in my tracks. Upon me were visited thirty days of furious depression and paralyzing anxiety. But when my life restarted in July, my eye was good. I saw I had some important choices.

All my life I had been presented with choices that most people don't get to make: What suitable clothes would I like to wear? What nutritious food would I like to eat? What sports would I play? Where would I go to college? Where did I want to live? What kind of job would I take? How hard did I want to work?

Most of my choosing had been mindless. I did not consider at the time why I chose to goof off in school. I did not consider why I always turned away from one type of woman and chose another. Even though I was no businessman, I did not closely examine why I chose to start an advertising agency. I did not consider the effect of my choice of words on other people's feelings. I had been living not my freedom but my high-class necessities instead.

Suffering improved my vision. After June 2004, I was able to see my choices, even if — like the prisoner — I had constraints. Looking back, it appears to me that I made seven good enough choices then and in the years that followed:

1. My first choice was to suffer better, to remain
    present for my thirty days of misery. Although
    I thought about it, I chose not to kill myself
    (proof my suffering could have been worse)
    or self-medicate with alcohol. With the help
    of my friends, my therapist, and a couple of
    prescriptions, I walked through Hell and got
    nicely roasted. Some impurities were burned
    off.

    The experience of pain can itself be an
    analgesic. Surviving that trial gave me courage
    to face other trials. It also gave me compassion.
    I was greatly oppressed by my own thoughts for
    thirty days. Some people are greatly oppressed
    by their own thoughts *every* day.

2. My second choice was to close down my
    advertising agency in an orderly fashion rather
    than locking the door and tossing the keys into
    bankruptcy court. I cut expenses to the bone. I
    held a three-week office equipment yard sale
    to raise cash. I used that cash to hire a lawyer. I
    moved into a cabin behind a friend's house. I
    moved my agency onto the table in that cabin.
    I sold my unneeded possessions on eBay. I
    bluffed and pleaded with the agency's creditors,
    endured a few insults, and cut deals.

    Instead of focusing on "How do I get back
    on my feet?" I inverted the problem: "How do
    I avoid being pushed further down?" I spent no
    time trying to get new advertising clients, no

time allocating blame to others, and no time
trying to cover up the failure of my business,
or my own failure. I focused on removing the
biggest problem: the threat of business and
then personal bankruptcy.

3. My third good enough choice was to start a new
    business rather than go back to the work I had
    been doing. My recent, vivid experience with
    near bankruptcy had given me some ideas. I
    started a business-to-business collection agency.
    People were surprised.

    Collection work pays well, but I wasn't going
    to make a new career there. My eccentric
    choice of how to pay my bills was a bridge to
    a future I could not see. I did not yet know
    I wanted to be a writer. I only knew that if
    I continued to do what I *had* been doing, I
    would crash again. My unconscious was telling
    me that much. I had the common sense to pay
    attention.

4. My fourth choice was to try to turn the
    journaling I had begun during my bad month
    into a book about procrastination, one of my
    bad habits. It became this book.

    Writing this book was not pulling a rabbit
    out of a hat, which had always been my
    specialty. It was climbing a mountain and
    building a metal shed at the same time. A tall
    mountain. Once in a while the view was great,
    but usually I climbed in fog. For years.

Many entries in my journal are similar to this one from June 2006: "Write, damn you. Suffer legitimately." Hey, I get to be pompous — it's my journal. Still, you can see there were times I was not inspired.

Nevertheless, the book gradually became my work, and doing my work gradually crowded out shame, half-heartedness, and despair. It gave me gumption.

You have to find *your* work. It may not pay any bills, but it *will* make you wholehearted. That's how you know it's your work.

5.   My work hasn't paid any bills, so another good enough choice was to begin marketing consulting, which I enjoy and am good at. It *does* pay my bills, letting me do what I have to do: write.

6.   My sixth choice was to eliminate things that distracted me from writing and marketing consulting. I find small-time stock trading to be endlessly fascinating, despite the fact that I am lousy at it. It is as engrossing as gambling but slightly more respectable. I came to recognize it as avoidance of my legitimate work. I broke up with stock trading and got engaged to Vanguard index funds.

I gradually pulled my heart back from my unconscious drive to avoid my work. I stopped studying for a graduate degree. I stopped going to casinos. I stopped going to meetings.

I stopped reading the *Wall Street Journal*. I
stopped watching a lot of TV. I stopped
saying yes to everything. I stopped attending
networking lunches. I gave up three-hour
workouts, baking bread, shoppertainment,
cutting the lawn, playing golf, and going to bars.
I gave up big dramas, arguments, lost causes,
and other interesting distractions. I did my
work. I may have chosen right or I may have
chosen wrong, but I chose. I don't know where
this will take me, but I know I am going there
in one piece. I am no longer divided against
myself.

7.   My seventh choice was to be kind. Kind to
myself, my family, my friends, and all of us.
Everyone is struggling to do their best, to
be more than they are now, some against
intractable forces. I will suspend judgment. I
will be kind.

It all sounds so nice and neat in retrospect. I woke up from
a thirty-day nightmare and confidently built a new and better way to live. Nothing could be further from the truth. It
has been a decade of two steps forward, one step back. There
were aftershocks from my great depression of 2004. I have
been stuck for long periods. I didn't write a word in 2009. I
have been terribly lonely. I have whined like a spoiled child.

I treated some people poorly. I lost clients. I have been up in the middle of the night full of anxiety hundreds of times. My journal is full of self-flagellation and laments about my lack of productivity, grit, drive, willpower, gumption.

I have not been great over the last ten years, but I have been good enough. That's excellent in my book.

Tolstoy wrote that true life is lived when tiny changes occur. Try to do a little better every day. Try to grow a little every day. You will fail many days. Can you learn from that and try again the next day? Maintain a ratio of two steps forward, one step back and you will do fine. Or even one and $\frac{1}{100}^{\text{th}}$ steps forward, one step back.

It will take much longer than you would like. It will be hard before it is easy. It will be embarrassing before it becomes a source of legitimate pride. You will need courage, common sense, and resourcefulness in harness together. You will need gumption.

You will need courage to drag your weakness out into the sunlight, as Ann Richards did with alcoholism. That will increase your courage. Look head on at your weakness and you will know what needs to be done. Simple. Not easy.

You will not make things worse by guessing. You will emulate Billy Beane, no math major himself, and try to choose better using the facts that matter for your work. Like John Snow, you will make a map that shows you the force of things.

You will increase your courage by knowing, daring, and

bearing discomfort. You will translate uncertainty as best you can and dare to accept the risk inherent in becoming more than you are now. You will remember when to ask yourself: "What have I got to lose?"

Like Julia Hill, 180 feet up a redwood, you will persevere. As you bear up to legitimate suffering you will build your fortitude — a crucial step in becoming more than you are now.

You will put excellence before success. You will put the things you can control — such as your preparation — in your decision frame and leave what you can't control — outcome — to The Everlasting Force of Every Thing.

You will pull up the anchor before adding sail. *Carpe defectum*: Seize the lessons of failure, particularly your own.

You will search for the vital few facts, the 20 percent of things that cause 80 percent of results. You will do the simple but difficult work of learning to want things that make you more than you are now, not less.

You will search for the incentives that drive your behavior and the behavior of others. Able to follow the money trail, you will avoid wasting time and money with spoonbenders. You will bend no spoons yourself.

You will increase your resourcefulness as you improve your vision, work at being creative, and develop your Who-Howness. Like Steve Jobs, you will look outside yourself for proof that the thing you need to do can be done. Like Oskar Schindler, you will create a lifesaving story from the means at hand. Like Galileo, you will check with people you trust and, once convinced of the worth of your ideas, you will stand behind them.

You will pursue your goals with passion. That is to say, you will suffer legitimately for your own redemption, for your own freedom, to be more than you are now.

You will be a scientist. You will follow Richard Feynman's example and be curious, diligent, and, if necessary, a bit irritating in your search for the truth, for the force of things. Knowing comes at a high price, but guessing is exorbitant.

In the ongoing fight for your own freedom, you won't always win, so try like hell to do what Ann Richards did. Find the fun in the fight. Go ahead and laugh at your ridiculous self. While moving forward.

As you think more about the choices you make, the workings of your own mind will become a topic of endless interest and importance. Without planning to, you will become a philosopher, concerning yourself with internal as opposed to external things.

As the philosopher Arthur Schopenhauer wrote, this may not make you a penny, but it *will* spare you the expense of seeking bad company and costly luxuries out of boredom.

As a philosopher, you will decide for yourself what you value. You will detach yourself from the world of "getting and spending," as Wordsworth called it, and use your time trying to acquire what is truly valuable.

As you grow your courage, resourcefulness, and common sense, you will grow your character. Now the secret that you knew all along: Gumption is character, the most important force of things in your life, the only force of things under your complete control.

As your character strengthens, your habits will improve. As your habits improve, your character will strengthen. A virtuous cycle. It also works in reverse.

Before you can do what you must do, when it ought to be done, you have to choose what that will be. Lose sixty pounds? Save for retirement? Get sober? Get organized? Change your career? Finish that screenplay? Clean up your neighborhood? Love yourself wholeheartedly? Love someone else wholeheartedly?

Those are important details, but they are details. Your real choice is this: Will you live your necessities or live your freedom?

All creatures live according to their necessities. Only people have the capacity to live into their freedom. People can make brave choices and accept the consequences. Simple. Not easy. Lifelong work. My lifelong work. *Your* lifelong work.

Lastly, friend: You were put here by The Everlasting Force of Every Thing to govern yourself reasonably. Nothing is more reasonable than to try your very best to take unreasonable joy in life. No matter where you're sitting, it's quite a show.

Go ahead now, astonish us.

Bonus *Gumptionade* material — including deleted sections, interactive worksheets, and a poster of Thomas Huxley's "the most valuable result of all education" quote — is available free at *www.gumptionade.com/readers-bonus*.

APPENDIX

GUMPTION CHECKLIST

COURAGE

☐ Choose excellence over success.
☐ Translate uncertainty into risk.
☐ Suffer better.

RESOURCEFULNESS

☐ Look for the force of things.
☐ Pull up the anchor before you add sail.
☐ Frame your decisions.

COMMON SENSE

☐ No spoonbending.
☐ Know your mind.
☐ Be less wrong.

GUMPTIONWORK

MY VITAL FEW FACTS
FROM *GUMPTIONADE*

You can do this better online:
www.gumptionade.com/extra-credit

Write down four or five important points from this book, if you please:

1. _____
2. _____
3. _____
4. _____
5. _____

If you could pick only one to remember, which would it be?

This is your vital fact, the 20 percent of what you got out of *Gumptionade* that will give you 80 percent of the benefit. Act on this and you will be more than you are now. A lot more.

ACKNOWLEDGMENTS

I would like to thank my first readers, particularly my wife Doralina, my son Jack O'Connor, Jill Piper, David Carlson, Susie Carlson, Bob Miller, Bill Walker, Richard Worth, Peter Mudd, Donna Kehoe, Richard Smoley, Peter Salisbury, Michele Matrisciani, Ellen Neuborne, Robin Wilson, Jim Anglin, Marion Kello, and Keith Parsons. Their advice and encouragement were important.

Thanks also to my editors, Jane Friedman, Beth Rashbaum, and Rachel Burd. They brought professionalism to *Gumptionade*. Thank you, Bristol Bell, for helping me push it over the finish line.

I could not have written this book without the positive influence on my life of the aforementioned Bill Walker, Jungian mystic and wise counselor.

I wish I could show this book to Bob and Dorothy.

NOTES

Front Material

1 **"Perhaps the most valuable result of all education…"** Thomas Huxley *Science & Education, Essays by Thomas Huxley* (1877) (The Project Gutenberg eBook #7150,2012) Essay XVI—Technical Education.

Introduction

2 **"Why don't they pass a constitutional amendment…?"** Professor Boerner's Explorations, http://www.boerner.net/jboerner/?p=14991. Accessed November 11, 2014.

3 **"If you are going to repair a motorcycle…"** Robert Pirsig, *Zen and the Art of Motorcycle Maintenance* (New York: William Morrow & Company, 1974), 303.

Section I : Gumption

Chapter 1: Buckets of Gumption

4 **"We had a pretty loud bang":** Gene Kranz, *Failure Is Not an Option* (New York: Berkley Books, 2000), 311.

5 **…pushed around by unidentified forces:** Ibid. 312.

6   She created her first political platform: Jan Reid, *Let the People In: The Life and Times of Ann Richards* (Austin: University of Texas Press, 2012), 28–29.

7   "...some of my finest drinking companions among them": Ann Richards, at the Celebration of Recovery (speech, Dallas, Texas, on September 29, 1995).

8   "We had to do it..." Reid, *Let the People In*, 112.

9   "You don't have to feel bad when you are drunk": Richards (speech, September 29, 1995).

10   "...everyone I ran with drank; I wasn't different": Steve Young, *Ann Richards: In Her Own Words*; available at http://www.huffingtonpost.com/steve-young/ann-richards-in-her own w_b_29/51.html, posted September 19, 2006, accessed July 6, 2014.

11   "There was no way I could survive it": Anne Richards with Peter Knobler, *Straight from the Heart: My Life in Politics and Other Places* (New York: Simon & Schuster 1989), 206

12   ...generated more non-tax revenue for the state than all previous treasurers combined: *A Guide to the Ann W. Richards Papers, Part 10. Treasury Papers, 1983–2000*. Brisco Center for American History, University of Texas at Austin.

13   "He was born with a silver foot in his mouth": "*Great Texas Women. Ann Richards/Texas Governor, 1933–2006*," University of Texas at Austin, *http://www.americanrhetoric.com/speeches/annrichards1988dnc.htm*. Keynote address to the Democratic National Convention, Atlanta, Georgia, July 18–21, 1988. Accessed 02/10/2014.

14   She also attended AA meetings...: Molly Ivins, "A-men. A-women. A-Ann. 10 years difference, and Ann Richards could've been president," *The Texas Observer*, October 6, 2006. *http://www.texasobserver.org/2309-a-men-a-women-a-ann-10-years-difference-and-ann-richards-couldve-been-president/*. Accessed July 5, 2014.

15   Ann Richards was the first governor to name significant numbers of minorities: "About Texas Gov. Ann Richards," Democratic Party of Collin County, Website: http://www.collindems.us/component/content/article/22/135-about-texas-gov-ann-richards.html Accessed July 5, 2014.

16   ... the boom that occurred years later. *http://www.collindems.us/component/content/article/22/135-about-texas-gov-ann-richards.html* ibid. Accessed July 5, 2014.

17   "We're all better than we think we are." Richards, speech, Dallas, Texas, September 29, 1995.

18   Since then, the A's have won 1,484 games. 1998–2014 seasons.

19   The New York Mets paid more than twice as much. *http://www*
.stevetheump.com/Payrolls.htm. Accessed October 20, 2014.

CHAPTER 2: GUMPTION IS COURAGE

20   "There was no courage in their taking such risks, just ignorance."
Nassim Taleb, *Fooled By Randomness* (New York: Random House, 2004).

21   "Sapere aude." Emmanuel Kant essay, What Is Enlightenment?

22   Hill bore the discomfort of freezing rain, forty-miles-per-hour
winds, and insomnia-inducing nocturnal squirrels. Julia Butterfly Hill,
The Legacy of Luna (San Francisco: Harper, 2000), 137.

CHAPTER 3: GUMPTION IS RESOURCEFULNESS

23   "...What we need is to use what we have." Basil S. Walsh http://www
.inspirationalstories.com/quotes/t/basil-s-walsh/. Accessed March 13, 2015.

24   "I could see what the future of computing was destined to be."
Walter Isaacson, *Steve Jobs* (New York: Simon & Schuster, 2011), 97.

25   "They were copier-heads who had no cluc what a computer could
do." Isaacson, *Steve Jobs*, 98.

26   ...a plastic bag, a sock, and a hose from one of the crew's pressure
suits. Gene Kranz, *Failure Is Not an Option* (New York: Berkley Books,
2000), 328.

27   "Galileo soon began to have doubts about this [heliocentric]
orthodoxy, which he aired in conversation with friends." Adam Gopnick
"Moon Man: What Galileo Saw," *The New Yorker*, February 11, 2013.

28   Wilbur Wright, co-owner of a bicycle shop, wrote to the
Smithsonian Institution in 1899. Wikipedia contributors, "Wright
brothers," Wikipedia, The Free Encyclopedia; http://en.wikipedia.org/w/
index.php?title=Wright_brothers&oldid=620917880. Accessed August 22,
2014.

29   What was lacking, what was crucial, was stability. Lawrence
Goldstone, *Birdmen: The Wright Brothers, Glenn Curtiss, and the Battle to
Control the Skies* (New York: Ballantine Books, 2014), 54–55.

30 "Perhaps the most challenging turnaround was accepting the need for assistance and help." Roger Epstein, "Buzz Aldrin: Down to Earth," *Psychology Today*, May 1, 2001; *http://www.psychologytoday.com/articles/200105/buzz-aldrin-down-earth* Accessed January 8, 2014.

CHAPTER 4: GUMPTION IS COMMON SENSE

31 "Philosophy is common sense with big words." James Madison; GoodReads.com; https://www.goodreads.com/quotes/6389-philosophy-is-common-sense-with-big-words. Accessed September 16, 2014.

32 What are the chances of a false positive on this test for someone with no known risk factors for AIDS? Gerd Gigerenzer, *Calculated Risks* (New York: Simon & Schuster, 2002), 125.

33 Americans with high stress from debt problems have heart attacks at twice the rate of those reporting low debt-related stress. Jeanine Aversa, "Stress over debt taking toll on health," *USA Today*, June 9, 2008. *http://usatoday30.usatoday.com/news/health/2008-06-09-debt-stress_N.htm.* Accessed August 19, 2014.

34 "Feynman is becoming a real pain." James Gleik, "Richard Feynman Dead at 69; Leading Theoretical Physicist," *New York Times*, February 17, 1988. *http://www.nytimes.com/1988/02/17/obituaries/richard-feynman-dead-at-69-leading-theoretical-physicist.html.* Accessed July 8, 2014.

35 NASA misunderstood commonly accepted measures of risk... Gleik. Ibid.

CHAPTER 5: GUMPTION IS NOT THIS

36 ...Pirsig writes of the things that halt progress for amateurs repairing their own motorcycles... Robert Pirsig, *Zen and the Art of Motorcycle Maintenance* (New York: William Morrow & Company, 1974), 305–26.

37 "Genius does what it must and talent does what it can." Robert Bulwer-Lytton, 1st Earl of Lytton, English dramatist, novelist, and politician (1803–73) *http://en.wikiquote.org/wiki/Robert_Bulwer-Lytton,_1st_Earl_of_Lytton.* Retrieved August 13, 2014.

38 "...these execrable eccentricities of instinct and conduct are only the evidences of genius, not the creators of it." Mark Twain, *The Late Ben Franklin*, 1870, quoted in *Blooms Classic Critical Views: Ben Franklin*, Edited by Harold Bloom (New York: InfoBase Publishing, 2008), 56.

39 Pauling was..."arguably the world's greatest quack." Paul Offit, "The Vitamin Myth: Why We Think We Need Supplements," *The Atlantic*, July 19, 2013; *http://www.theatlantic.com/health/archive/2013/07/the-vitamin-myth-why-we-think-we-need-supplements/277947/*.

SECTION II: HOW TO BE COURAGEOUS

CHAPTER 6: KNOW WHAT COURAGE IS FOR

40 "Everybody has a plan until they get punched in the mouth." Mike Berardino, "Mike Tyson explains one of his most famous quotes," *Sun-Sentinel*, November 9, 2012. http://articles.sun-sentinel.com/2012-11-09/sports/sfl-mike-tyson-explains-one-of-his-most-famous-quotes-2012110. Accessed March 13, 2015

41 "Yes Ma'am, but there are some things'll scare you so bad you hurt yourself." Molly Ivins, "The Fun's in the Fight," *Mother Jones* (May/June 1993).

42 "A mechanic who has a big ego to defend is at a terrific disadvantage." Pirsig, *Zen and the Art of Motorcycle Maintenance*, 314.

43 "It's either a prize carrot or a stunted gourd!" Edmond Rostand, *Cyrano de Bergerac*, Literary Classics Collection, G Books, 2011 (Kindle Edition: loc 990).

44 "Why can't I be both?" William B. Irvine, *A Guide to the Good Life: The Ancient Art of Stoic Joy* (Oxford: Oxford University Press, 2009), 255.

45 "...a reservoir of good spirits." Pirsig, *Zen and the Art of Motorcycle Maintenance*, 305.

46 "I shall keep watching myself continually..." Wikisource contributors, 'Moral letters to Lucilius/Letter 83', Wikisource, 6 October 2014, 18:53 UTC, http://en.wikisource.org/w/index.php?title=Moral_letters_to_Lucilius/Letter_83&oldid=5072621. Accessed 18 December 2014.

CHAPTER 7: PUT EXCELLENCE BEFORE SUCCESS

47 "…we have a right to our labor, but not to the fruits of our labor." Steven Pressfield, *The War of Art: Break through the Blocks and Win Your Inner Creative Battles* (New York: Black Irish Entertainment, 2012), 161.

48 …the now forgotten Francis Beaumont and John Fletcher. Wikipedia contributors, "Shakespeare's reputation," Wikipedia, The Free Encyclopedia; *http://en.wikipedia.org/w/index.php?title=Shakespeare%27s_reputation&oldid=621047186.* Accessed August 23, 2014.

49 "There are many people, particularly in sports, who think that success and excellence are the same thing." Joe Paterno, *https://www.goodreads.com/quotes/tag/excellence.* Accessed August 23, 2014.

50 "…any concern for the safety and well-being of Sandusky's victims until after Sandusky's arrest." Press Release, *Remarks of Louis Freeh in Conjunction with Announcement of Publication of Report Regarding the Pennsylvania State University*, Philadelphia, PA, July 12, 2012, 4. *http://progress.psu.edu/assets/content/Press_Release_07_12_12.pdf.* Accessed August 23, 2014.

51 "See how many qualities there are which could be yours at this moment." Marcus Aurelius, *Meditations* (New York: Penguin Books, 2005), 44–45.

CHAPTER 8: TRANSLATE UNCERTAINTY INTO RISK

52 …return to London with Swedish timber, hemp, and bar iron. Chris Evans, Owen Jackson, and Goran Ryden, *Economic History Review*, LV, 4 (Oxford: Blackwell Publishers, 2002), 642–65.

53 There is a tool for measuring uncertainty. It is called statistics. Of course that tool is more accurately called actuarial science, but actuarial science is outside of the scope of this book.

54 Insist upon actual frequency to better weigh risk. Gerd Gigerenzer, *Calculated Risks* (New York: Simon & Schuster, 2002), 205.

55 "Statistical thinking will one day be as necessary for efficient citizenship as the ability to read and write." H. G. Wells, as quoted in Gigerenzer, *Calculated Risks*, 23

56 … the risk of smoking, which costs women an average of 4.6 years of life. Scott Plous, *The Psychology of Judgment and Decision Making* (New York: McGraw-Hill, 1993), 138.

57 ...the risk of living near a nuclear power plant, less dangerous than riding a bicycle. Ibid. 140.

58 Statistics show that disease causes about sixteen times as many deaths as accidents... Sarah Lichtenstein, Paul Slovic, et al., "Judged Frequency of Lethal Events," *Journal of Experimental Psychology: Human Learning and Memory* 4 no. 6 (November 1978), 551–78; *http://psycnet.apa.org/journals/xlm/4/6/551/*. Cited by Elizier Yudkowsky "Availability" at Less Wrong—A community blog devoted to refining the art of rationality. http://lesswrong.com/lw/j5/availability/. Accessed August 23, 2014.

59 You are about one hundred times more likely to be killed by lightning than you are to win a million-dollar lottery prize. "Lifetime odds of death for selected causes, United States, 2009," National Safety Council, *Injury Facts, 2013 Edition; http://www.nsc.org/news_resources/injury_and_death_statistics/Documents/Injury_Facts_43.pdf*. Accessed March 4, 2014.

60 He says now that he "made a mistake in presuming" that financial firms could regulate themselves. "25 People to Blame for the Financial Crisis: The good intentions, bad managers and greed behind the meltdown," *Time; http://content.time.com/time/specials/packages/article/0,28804, 1877351_1877350_1877331, 00.html#ixzz2vICCHbNH*. Accessed March 6, 2014.

61 "...the probability of failure combined with the consequences to human health and safety if that failure were to occur." "The New Orleans Hurricane Protection System: What Went Wrong and Why—A Report by the American Society of Civil Engineers Hurricane Katrina Review Panel" 2007. *http://www.asce.org/uploadedfiles/publications/asce_news/2009/04_april/erpreport.pdf*. Accessed September 24, 2014.

62 Helmets are the main reason there are so many head injuries in football. *http://profootballtalk.nbcsports.com/2012/12/04/hines-ward-if-you-want-to-prevent-concussions-take-the-helmet-off/*. Accessed March 18, 2015.

63 The rate of death from skydiving accidents remains stable. Lessons to be Learned—The 2012 Fatality Summary. *http://parachutistonline.com/feature/lessons-to-be-learned*. Accessed September 9, 2015.

64 Smoking increases the risk of... Centers for Disease Control and Prevention website http://www.cdc.gov/tobacco/data_statistics/fact_sheets/health_effects/effects_cig_smoking/. Accessed July 25, 2014.

65   Approximately 5 percent of the general adult population has a
sex addiction. Timothy Fond, M.D., "Understanding and Managing
Compulsive Sexual Behaviors," *Psychiatry* 3 no. 11 (November 2006),
51–58; *http://www.ncbi.nlm.nih.gov/pmc/articles/PMC2945841/#B8*.
Accessed July 26, 2014.

66   Women who identified their work as highly stressful were 40
percent more likely… Cesar Chelala, "What's the point in working
yourself to death?" *The Japan Times*, January 7, 2013; *http://www
.japantimes.co.jp/opinion/2013/01/07/commentary/world-commentary/whats-
the-point-in-working-yourself-to-death/#.U_jVVPmwKHt*. Accessed July 26,
2014.

67   …reduce their returns by about 4 percent annually versus investors
who buy and hold low-cost mutual funds. Brad M. Barber, Yi-Tsung
Lee, Yu-Jane Liu, et al., "Just How Much Do Individual Investors Lose by
Trading?" *The Review of Financial Studies* 22 no. 2 (2009).

68   Obesity increases the risk of… Specific disease statistics citations
a–f below are from: Harvard School of Public Health, Obesity Prevention
Source, "Health Risks," *http://www.hsph.harvard.edu/obesity-prevention-
source/obesity-consequences/health-effects/#references*. Accessed July 25,
2014:

69   a. Diabetes… D. P. Guh, W. Zhang, N. Bansback, et al, "The
incidence of co-morbidities related to obesity and overweight: a
systematic review and meta-analysis," *BMC Public Health* 9 (2009), 88.

70   b. Heart Disease… R. P. Bogers, W. J. Bemelmans, R. T.
Hoogenveen, et al, "Association of overweight with increased risk
of coronary heart disease partly independent of blood pressure and
cholesterol levels: a meta-analysis of 21 cohort studies including more
than 300,000 persons," *Archives of Internal Medicine*. 167 (2007),
1720–8.

71   c. Stroke… P. Strazzullo, L. D'Elia, G. Cairella, et al., "Excess
body weight and incidence of stroke: meta-analysis of prospective
studies with 2 million participants." *Stroke*, 41 (2010), e418–26.

72   d. Depression… F. S. Luppino, L. M. de Wit, P. F. Bouvy, et al,
"Overweight, obesity, and depression: a systematic review and meta-
analysis of longitudinal studies," *Archives of General Psychiatry* 67
(2010), 220–9.

73   e. Asthma… D. A. Beuther, E. R, Sutherland, "Overweight,
obesity, and incident asthma: a meta-analysis of prospective
epidemiologic studies," *Am J Respiratory Critical Care Med* 175 (2007),
661–6.

74   **f. Alzheimer's…** M. A. Beydoun, H. A. Beydoun, Y. Wang, "Obesity and central obesity as risk factors for incident dementia and its subtypes: a systematic review and meta-analysis," *Obesity Review* 9 (2008), 204–18.

75   **g. Getting ten types of cancer…** G. K. Reeves, K. Pirie, V. Beral, et al., Million Women Study Collaboration. "Cancer incidence and mortality in relation to body mass index in the Million Women Study: cohort study,"*The BMJ* 335 no. 7630 (December 1, 2007), 1134; Epub: November 6, 2007; *http://www.ncbi.nlm.nih.gov/pubmed/17986716.* Accessed July 25, 2014.

76   **25 percent of women who have more than seven alcoholic drinks per week are considered to be dependent on alcohol (fourteen drinks per week for men).** *Drinking Levels Defined,* National Institute on Alcohol Abuse and Alcoholism, *http://www.niaaa.nih.gov/alcohol-health/ overview-alcohol-consumption/moderate-binge-drinking.* Accessed July 25, 2014.

77   **FindingPneumo exercise** based on Gerd Gigerenzer, *Calculated Risks* (New York: Simon & Schuster, 2002), 125.

Chapter 9: Suffer Better

78   **"Where is it written that you're supposed to be happy all the time?"** Transcript of May 23, 2013, "What We Nurture" interview with Krista Tippett from *On Being* Web site; *http://www.onbeing.org/program/what-we-nurture-with-sylvia-boorstein/transcript/5581.* Accessed March 13, 2014.

79   **"The memory of pain can itself be a painkiller."** Paul Theroux, "The Best Year of My Life," *The New Yorker,* November 14, 2005; *http:// www.newyorker.com/magazine/2005/11/14/the-best-year-of-my-life.* Accessed July 25, 2014.

80   **"…whipping post."** Song written by Greg Allman, performed by The Allman Brothers Band.

Section III: How to Be Resourceful

Chapter 10: Look for the Force of Things

81 "Assuredly the reason is that the earth draws it." William Stukeley, *Memoirs of Sir Isaac Newton's Life* from Wikipedia contributors, "Isaac Newton," Wikipedia, The Free Encyclopedia, *http://en.wikipedia.org/w/index.php?title=Isaac_Newton&oldid=622141882*. Accessed June 19, 2014.

82 Seneca wrote that drunkenness is insanity purposefully assumed: Seneca Letters LXXXIII: *On Drunkenness*, TheStoicLife.org, *https://sites.google.com/site/thestoiclife/the_teachers/seneca/letters/083*. Accessed September 10, 2015.

83 "There was a child went forth": Walt Whitman, *Leaves of Grass* (New York: Andrew Rome, 1855) 90.

84 … your childhood remains at the core: W. Hugh Missildine, M.D., *Your Inner Child of the Past* (New York: Pocket Books, 1963), 41.

85 "…a feeling the child has of being isolated and helpless in a potentially hostile world." Karen Horney, M.D., *Our Inner Conflicts: A Constructive Theory of Neurosis* (New York: W.W. Norton, 1945), 41.

86 This is how adults behave! Missildine, *Your Inner Child of the Past*, 188.

87 "…lasting character trends which become part of his personality." Horney, *Our Inner Conflicts*, 42

88 "When I was a child, I talked like a child, I thought like a child, I reasoned like a child." St. Paul, *Letter to the Corinthians*, 1 Corinthians 13. New International Version of the Bible *http://biblehub.com/1_corinthians/13-11.htm*. Accessed September 25, 2014.

89 The Adverse Childhood Experiences (ACE) Study. Robert Anda, MD, MS, "The Health and Social Impact of Growing Up with Adverse Childhood Experiences: The Human and Economic Costs of the Status Quo." Dr. Anda was the co-principal investigator of the Adverse Childhood Experiences (ACE) study. *http://acestudy.org/files/Review_of_ACE_Study_with_references_summary_table_2_.pdf*. Accessed April 24, 2014.

90 … normal stress response system becomes hyperactive and stays that
way. Center on the Developing Child at Harvard University, "Excessive
Stress Disrupts the Architecture of the Developing Brain: Working Paper
3"; http://developingchild.harvard.edu/resources/reports_and_working_
papers/working_papers/wp3/. Accessed August 24, 2014.

91 …anger, depression, hypervigilance, and avoidant behaviors.
Wikipedia contributors, "Posttraumatic stress disorder," Wikipedia,
The Free Encyclopedia; http://en.wikipedia.org/w/index
.php?title=Posttraumatic_stress_disorder&oldid=622426266. Accessed
August 23, 2014.

92 … cutting the lawn with a straight razor. Chuck Squatriglia, "Dr.
Allen Wheelis—Acclaimed Writer," *San Francisco Chronicle*, June 24,
2007; *http://www.sfgate.com/bayarea/article/Dr-Allen-Wheelis-acclaimed-
writer-2584671.php*. Accessed July 1, 2013.

93 "What has made my father's voice so irresistible all these years…"
Allen Wheelis, *How People Change* (New York: Harper Colophon Books,
1973), 83.

94 …harshly criticized by the American College of Radiology and the
Society of Breast Imaging: Bradford Pearson, "Study: Mammograms
Do Not Save Lives," *Healthcare Daily*, February 2, 2014 *http://healthcare*
.dmagazine.com/2014/02/14/study-mammograms-do-not-save-lives/.
Accessed March 27, 2014.

Chapter 11: Pull Up the Anchor
Before You Add Sail

95 "Man muss immer umkehren" (Invert) "Wikipedia contributors,
"Carl Gustav Jacob Jacobi," Wikipedia, The Free Encyclopedia,
http://en.wikipedia.org/w/index.php?title=Carl_Gustav_Jacob_
Jacobi&oldid=626833898. Accessed March 18, 2015.

96 "…pick the ten or fifteen worst performers and take them out of
the sample, and work with the residual." Frederick F. Reichheld, *The
Loyalty Effect* (Boston: Harvard Business School Press, 1996), 190.

97 "I hate to lose worse than anyone…" http://www.saturdaydownsouth
.com/alabama-football/encouraging-bear-bryant-quotes/. Accessed March
13, 2015.

98   "The probable cause of this accident was…" National
Transportation Safety Board, "Aircraft Accident Report May 25, 1979,"
December 21, 1979; *http://libraryonline.erau.edu/online-full-text/ntsb/
aircraft-accident-reports/AAR79-17.pdf* Accessed August 23, 2014.

99   There were less than two hundred U.S. commercial airline
fatalities in the ten years ending with 2012: Joshua Freed and Scott
Mayerowitz, "U.S. commercial airlines have safest decade ever,"
Associated Press, January 1, 2012, San Francisco Chronicle; *http://www.
sfgate.com/nation/article/U-S-commercial-airlines-have-safest-decade-
ever-2435203.php*. Accessed August 23, 2014.

100   A recent study in the *Journal of Patient Safety* estimated there are
over 200,000 preventable deaths of hospital patients *every year.* John
T. James, "A New, Evidence-based Estimate of Patient Harms Associated
with Hospital Care, *Journal of Patient Safety* 9, issue 3 (September 2013),
122–28; *http://journals.lww.com/journalpatientsafety/Fulltext/2013/09000/A_
New,_Evidence_based_Estimate_of_Patient_Harms.2.aspx*. Accessed on
March 31, 2014.

101   …might cast a spell of fatal dread—panic—into humans… Joseph
Campbell, *The Hero with a Thousand Faces*, 3rd ed. (Novato, CA: New
World Library, 2008), 66–7

102   King Lear: When were you wont to be so full of songs, sirrah?
William Shakespeare, *King Lear* (New York: Dover Publications, 1994).
Act I, Scene 4.

CHAPTER 12: FRAME YOUR DECISIONS

103   The A299 was considered too complicated to fly safely Philip
Meilinger, "When the Fortress Went Down," *Air Force Magazine* 87,
no. 10 (October 2004), 78–82. Cited by Atul Gawande in *The Checklist
Manifesto* (New York: Metropolitan Books, 2009), 32–3.

104   …the Douglas DB-1, which later proved unsatisfactory for combat
operations: Ibid.

105   The B-17 achieved iconic status because…Wikipedia contributors,
"Boeing B-17 Flying Fortress," Wikipedia, The Free Encyclopedia,
http://en.wikipedia.org/w/index.php?title=Boeing_B-17_Flying_
Fortress&oldid=621927748. Accessed August 24, 2014.

106   Simple formulas are more accurate than expert opinion, particularly in low-validity environments. Daniel Kahneman, *Thinking Fast and Slow* (New York: Farrar, Straus & Giroux, 2011), 222–3.

SECTION IV: HOW TO HAVE COMMON SENSE

CHAPTER 13: NO SPOONBENDING

107   "We have now sunk to a depth at which restatement of the obvious…" George Orwell's January 1939 review published in *Adlephi*, of Bertrand Russell's book *Power: A New Social Analysis*; http://www.lehman .edu/deanhum/philosophy/BRSQ/06may/orwell.htm. Accessed March 13, 2015.

108   Over one hundred million people in the United States go on a diet in any given year. ABC News Staff, "100 Million Dieters, $20 Billion: The Weight-Loss Industry by the Numbers," Posted May 8, 2012; *http:// abcnews.go.com/Health/100-million-dieters-20-billion-weight-loss-industry/ story?id=16297197*. Accessed August 24, 2014.

109   …the illusion of painless, convenient change. Keith Girard, "Startup Stories: Challenging Diet Industry Giants with a Computer," allBusiness.com, undated; *http://www.allbusiness.com/company-activities- management/company-structures/5963512-1.html*. Accessed August 24, 2014.

110   …add the lost weight back in a year or two. Rena R. Wing, Ph.D., Deborah F. Tate, Ph.D., Amy A. Gorin, Ph.D., et al., "A Self-Regulation Program for Maintenance of Weight Loss," *New England Journal of Medicine*, 355:1563–1571, October 12, 2006.

111   …"the laborious adaptations and manifold disappointments that accompany any sort of significant personal progress." C. G. Jung, *AION: Researches into the Phenomenology of the Self* (Princeton, NJ: Princeton University Press, 1978), 34.

112   They replace snake handling with fire walking… Micki McGee, *Self Help, Inc.: Makeover Culture in American Life* (Oxford: Oxford University Press, 2005), 60.

113   Magic advises opening up your channel… Shakti Gawain, *Living in the Light* (Mill Valley, CA: Whatever Publishing, 1986), 142. Direct quote cited by McGee, *Self Help, Inc.*, on page 72.

114 **"Prepare your wish list to the universe"**: Sarah Ban Breathnach, *Simple Abundance: A Daybook of Comfort and Joy* (New York: Grand Central Publishing, 1994). Cited by McGee *Self-Help, Inc.*, page 164.

115 **...life is like managing an investment portfolio.** McGee, *Self-Help, Inc.*, 69.

116 **...emotional bank account:** FranklinCovey Blog "Emotional Bank Account," *http://www.franklincovey.com/blog/tag/emotional-bank-account.* Accessed September 25, 2014

117 **Physician Atul Gawande writes about the yawning gap...** Atul Gawande, "The Checklist," *The New Yorker*, December 10, 2007.

CHAPTER 14: KNOW YOUR MIND

118 **Philosophers and scientists since Plato have recognized...** Leonard Mlodinow, *Subliminal: How Your Unconscious Mind Rules Your Behavior* (New York: Pantheon Books, 2012), 96.

119 **"The most decisive qualities in a person..."** C. G. Jung, *AION: Researches into the Phenomenology of the Self* (Princeton, NJ: Princeton University Press 1978), 5.

120 **About a third of your brain is devoted to vision.** Mlodinow, *Subliminal*, 35.

121 **Major league baseball umpires expand the strike zone for veteran pitchers.** Phil Birnbaum, "Do Umpires Discriminate in Favor of Veterans?" *Sabermetric Research*, August 1, 2011; reprinted on blog *http://blog.philbirnbaum.com/2011/08/do-umpires-discriminate-in-favor-of.html.* Accessed August 24, 2014.

122 **Later rated these students subsequently also received higher grades than the other students:** Mlodinow, *Subliminal*, 113.

123 **...and be generally happier than people with average looks.** Dion, K, E. Berscheid, E. Walster, "What Is Beautiful Is Good," *Journal of Personality and Social Psychology* 24 no. 3 (December 1972), 285–90.

124 **There's a lot going on there.** Mlodinow, *Subliminal*. 33–4.

125 **"Contempt is the weapon of the weak..."** Alice Miller, *Prisoners of Childhood* (New York: Basic Books, 1981), 69.

126 ...projection of fear and anger onto a scapegoat group by economically endangered whites. C. I. Hovland, R. R. Sears, "Minor studies of aggression: VI. Correlation of lynchings with economic indices," *Journal of Psychology: Interdisciplinary and Applied* 9 (1940), 301–10.

CHAPTER 15: BE LESS WRONG

127 **Less Wrong.** This chapter title was inspired by LessWrong.com, a community blog devoted to refining the art of human rationality. *http:// lesswrong.com/*

128 **Sometimes you feel like a nut...** Wikipedia contributors, "Leon Carr," Wikipedia, The Free Encyclopedia, *http://en.wikipedia.org/w/index. php?title=Leon_Carr&oldid=643297701.* Accessed March 12, 2015.

129 **What percentage of UN member states are African?** Daniel Kahneman, *Thinking Fast and Slow* (New York: Farrar, Straus & Giroux, 2011), 119–20.

130 **People are anchored to their own name.** Leonard Mlodinow, *Subliminal: How Your Unconscious Mind Rules Your Behavior* (New York: Pantheon Books, 2012), 19.

131 **Monkey is in danger...** Pirsig, *Zen and the Art of Motorcycle Maintenance* 303.

132 **Then you rejected a guaranteed $500.** Kahneman, *Thinking Fast and Slow*, 280.

133 **If you are normal, you will take risks to avoid a loss...** [Loss Aversion]. Scott Plous, *The Psychology of Judgment and Decision Making* (New York: McGraw-Hill, 1993), 96.

134 **Which of them is more likely to risk the drive?** [Chasing Losses]. Kahneman, *Thinking Fast and Slow*, 343.

135 **...evolution designed your brain for survival, not self-awareness.** Mlodinow, *Subliminal*, 194.

136 **Randomness does not look random.** Nassim Taleb, *Fooled by Randomness* (New York: Random House, 2004), 54.

137 **...hindsight bias...** Scott Plous, *The Psychology of Judgment and Decision Making* (New York: McGraw-Hill, 1993), 138.

138 **...by purchasing eight of his Prince Castle five-spindle Multimixers?** Ray Kroc with Ronald Anderson, *Grinding It Out — The Making of McDonalds* (Chicago: Contemporary Books, 1977), 6.

139 ...a bright kid at Lakeside Middle School could learn computer programming. Stephan Manes, Paul Andrews, *Gates: How Microsoft's Mogul Reinvented an Industry and Made Himself the Richest Man in America* (Seattle: Cadwaller & Stern, 2013—Kindle Edition).

140 ...Kahneman cites a study showing that judges paroled significantly fewer prisoners in the hour before lunch. Kahneman, *Thinking Fast and Slow*, 44.

141 ...the budget for the project had been based on "unfounded optimism." Tony Capaccio, "Lockheed F-35 Overruns Top $1 Billion, Government Auditor Finds," March 20, 2012, *Bloomberg; http://www .bloomberg.com/news/2012-03-20/lockheed-f-35-overruns-top-1-billion-government-auditor-finds.html*. Accessed August 24, 2014.

142 The average cost overrun on defense acquisition contracts is 40 percent. David S. Christensen, "An Analysis of Cost Overruns on Defense Acquisition Contracts," *Project Management Journal* 3 (September, 1993), 43 48.

143 The Big Dig ... final bill was $22 billion. Joseph Lawler, "The Bigger Dig— Lessons on Expanding Infrastructure Projects from the State of Massachusetts," *The American Spectator*, February 13, 2009.

144 ..."spending more time stuck in traffic rather than less." Sean P. Murphy, "Big Dig pushes bottlenecks outward," *The Boston Globe/ boston.com*, November 16, 2008; *http://www.boston.com/news/local/ articles/2008/11/16/big_dig_pushes_bottlenecks_outward/?page=full*. Accessed August 24, 2014.

145 The Sydney Opera house...: Dr. Paol Canonico and Dr. Jonas Söderlund, "The Sydney Opera House—Stakeholder Management and Project Success," (*Project Management* 722G20: February 13, 2009); A case study. *http://www.iei.liu.se/fek/svp/723g18/case_material/1.111101/ SydneyOperaHouseProjectStudy.pdf*. Accessed April 20, 2014.

146 ...the continued good credit performance of subprime mortgage pools... "Housing Outlook," J.P. Morgan Research, June 17, 2005, as quoted in the anonymously written website *The Economics of Contempt* post titled "The Unofficial List of Pundits/Experts Who Were Wrong on the Housing Bubble," posted July 16, 2008; *http://economicsofcontempt .blogspot.com/2008/07/official-list-of-punditsexperts-who.html*. Accessed August 24, 2014.

147 ...Touch of Yogurt shampoo? Matt Haig, *Brand Failures: The Truth About the 100 Biggest Branding Mistakes of All Time* (Philadelphia: Kogan Page Business Books, 2003), 53.

148   *Cleopatra* — budgeted at $2 million 1963 dollars but costing $44 million... Stephen Simon, "The Soul of the Movies," December 15, 2010; theoldhollywood.com

149   **Waterworld**... *Wikipedia contributors, "Waterworld," Wikipedia, The Free Encyclopedia, http://en.wikipedia.org/w/index.php?title=Waterworld& oldid=650399523.* Accessed March 12, 2015.

150   United Artists' fiscal disaster Heaven's Gate... Wikipedia contributors, "Heaven's Gate (film)," Wikipedia, The Free Encyclopedia; *http://en.wikipedia.org/w/index.php?title=Heaven%27s_Gate_ (film)&oldid=622051119.* Accessed August 24, 2014.

151   The accuracy of her clear, vivid and recent memory is surprisingly poor. Mlodinow, *Subliminal*, 60–1.

152   Half of the discussion they did recall never actually occurred: I.M.L. Hunter, *Memory* (Middlesex, England, Penguin Books, 1964). Cited by Plous, *The Psychology of Judgment and Decision Making*, 37.

153   People and their behaviors are the easiest ingredients to remember: Ibid. 180.

154   Situational factors such as time pressure, temperature, and noise... Ibid. 180–1.

155   ...hold a pre-mortem..." Kahneman *Thinking Fast and Slow*; 264–5

156   "Every man carries with him the world in which he must live." F. Marion Crawford, *Cecilia: A Story of Modern Rome* from *The Complete Works of F. Marion Crawford*, vol 30 (New York: P. F. Collier & Son, 1902).

Section V: How to Go from Here

Chapter 16: Choose

157   "...then — however he choose — he is living his freedom." Allen Wheelis, *How People Change* (New York: Harper Colophon Books, 1973), 32.

158 "…getting and spending," as Wordsworth called it… William Wordsworth, "The World Is Too Much with Us: Late and Soon," *The Complete Poetical Works*, by William Wordsworth (London: Macmillan and Co., 1888). *http://www.bartleby.com/145/ww317.html*. Accessed September 29, 2014.

GLOSSARY

Creative Suffering Discomfort that makes you better than you were. For example, playing your piano scales or going jogging when you should, but really don't want to. (See also "Day Four.")

Day Four The moment when your enthusiasm for self-improvement is gone and things get hard. (See also "Creative Suffering.")

FindingPneumo A fictional disease used in this book to illustrate the hazards of the false positive.

Go Fever The top-down bias of a group toward consensus and forward movement without effective consideration of risk.

Gumptionade Thoughts and actions that boost your courage, resourcefulness, and common sense.

Invert A method for solving hard problems by turning them upside down.

Invisible Reference Points Ideas lodged in your mind that influence your thoughts and behavior without you being aware.

Kudos Congratulations.

Jack Tar A nickname for English sailors used primarily in the 19th century. (The name of Jack's bosun, Bill Bobstay, comes from the 1878 Gilbert and Sullivan operetta *H.M.S. Pinafore*. A bobstay is a part of the rigging of a ship.)

Law of the Vital Few Vilfredo Pareto's discovery, often called the 80/20 rule: Twenty percent of anything will produce eighty percent of the results.

Low-Validity Environment Early childhood, the stock market, first dates: environments likely to give unreliable information such as false positives.

Magoo My term for people who appear—even to themselves— successful, clever, and/or brave, but are actually blind to the real risks they are taking. The term originates with Quincy Magoo, the extremely nearsighted central character of the TV cartoon *The Famous Adventures of Mr. Magoo.*

Metal Shed My term for something you must do even though you did not realize just how difficult it would be when you agreed to do it. Metal Shed moments separate people who do what they say they will from everybody else. The term comes from my story about building a metal shed in Chapter 9 ("Suffer Better") of this book.

Psycho-logic My way of saying that important decisions can be driven by habit, intuition, and emotion, rather than logic. People are often not logical, they are *psycho-logical.*

Spoonbending Thrilling illusions that yield no meaningful outcome. ("Eat what you want and still lose weight.") Named for magician Uri Geller's trick of appearing to bend spoons with the power of his mind.

Spray 'n Change The type of plans and products we buy when we want shortcuts to our self-improvement goals. (See also "Go Fever" and "Spoonbending.")

The Child You Were Lasting character traits developed during your childhood (see also "Low-Validity Environment") that affect the way you behave and think now, usually without you being aware. (See also "Invisible Reference Points.")

The Force of Things How the universe works, including the universe inside your head. Usually invisible, especially the forces that affect human decision making.

Turkey Problem From a story of a turkey on a farm who liked how he was treated every day, until the day he became Thanksgiving dinner. Used to show the limits of inductive reasoning, which is deriving a general principle from specific observations.

WhoHowness My term for the skill of knowing who, how, and when to ask for help. A key aspect of resourcefulness.

Your Hairy Ancestor Instincts and behavior from humanity's collective evolutionary past that affect the way you behave and think, often without you being aware. (See also "Invisible Reference Points.")

BIBLIOGRAPHY

Aurelius, Marcus. *Meditations*. New York: Penguin Books, 2005

Campbell, Joseph. *The Hero with a Thousand Faces*. New York: Pantheon Books, 1949.

Feynman, Richard P. *"What Do You Care What Other People Think?"* New York: W.W. Norton, 1988

Gawande, Atul. *The Checklist Manifesto*. New York: Metropolitan Books, 2009.

Gigerenzer, Gerd. *Calculated Risks*. New York: Random House, 2002.

Gigerenzer, Gerd. *Risk Savvy: How to Make Good Decisions*. New York: Random House, 2004.

Hill, Julia Butterfly. *The Legacy of Luna*. New York: HarperCollins, 2000.

Horney, Karen, M.D. *Our Inner Conflicts*. New York: W. W. Norton & Company, 1945.

Irvine, William. *A Guide to the Good Life: The Ancient Art of Stoic Joy*. New York: Oxford University Press, 2009.

Isaacson, Walter. *Steve Jobs*. New York: Simon & Schuster, 2011

Jung, C.G. *Aion: Researches into the Phenomenology of the Self*. Princeton, NJ: Princeton University Press, 1959.

Kahneman, Daniel. *Thinking, Fast and Slow*. New York: Farrar, Straus and Giroux, 2011.

Kranz, Gene. *Failure Is Not an Option*. New York: Berkley Publishing Group, 2000.

McGee, Micki. *Self-Help, Inc.* New York: Oxford University Press, 2005.

Miller, Alice. *Prisoners of Childhood*. New York: Basic Books, 1981.

Missildine, W. Hugh, M.D. *Your Inner Child of the Past*. New York: Pocket Books, 1963.

Mlodinow, Leonard. *Subliminal: How Your Unconscious Mind Rules Your Behavior*. New York: Pantheon Books, 2012.

Osbon, Diane K.. *A Joseph Campbell Companion: Reflections on the Art of Living*. New York: HarperCollins, 1991.

Pirsig, Robert. *Zen and the Art of Motorcycle Maintenance: An Inquiry into Values*. New York: William Morrow & Company, Inc, 1974.

Plous, Scott. *The Psychology of Judgment and Decision Making*. New York: McGraw-Hill, 1993.

Pressfield, Steven. *The War of Art*. New York: Black Irish Entertainment, 2002.

Reichheld, Frederick. *The Loyalty Effect*. Watertown, MA: Harvard Business School Press, 1996.

Taleb, Nassim Nicholas. *Fooled by Randomness*. New York: Random House, 2004.

Taleb, Nassim Nicholas. *The Black Swan*. New York: Random House, 2007.

Wheelis, Allen. *How People Change*. New York: Harper Colophon, 1973.

INDEX